Remembering Our Home

Healing Hurts & Receiving Gifts from Conception to Birth

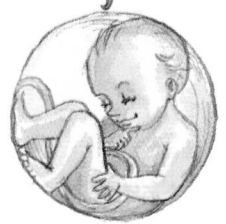

**Sheila Fabricant Linn
William Emerson
Dennis Linn
Matthew Linn, S.J.**

Illustrations by Francisco Miranda

Paulist Press
New York / Mahwah, New Jersey

Acknowledgments

We want to thank the following persons for their time and loving care in helping us with the manuscript for this book: Martha Backstrom, Patricia Berne & Lou Savary, Ray Castellino, Maria Esther Castillo, David Chamberlain, Kevin John Clark, Michael Clifford, Mary Ellen DeRosa, Millie Dosh, Bob & Ginny Flanagan, Margaret Grant, W. Joseph Hanss, John Rice, Peg Rubin, Doug Schoeninger, Bob Sears, S.J., Char Spade, Len Sperry, and Chris Wade.

The publisher gratefully acknowledges use of the following: excerpt from "Ode on Intimations of Immortality" from *The Complete Poetical Works of William Wordsworth* (London: Macmillan, 1888); boxes titled "Growth and Changes During Pregnancy" and "The Growth and Development of the Fetus" from American College of Obstetricians and Gynecologists, *Planning for Pregnancy, Birth, and Beyond*, 2nd ed., Washington, D.C. © ACOG, 1995, used with permission; photos of developing embryo during the first eight weeks of pregnancy, used courtesy of Carnegie Institution of Washington.

Book Design by Saija Autrand, Faces Type & Design

IMPRIMI POTEST:
D. Edward Mathie, S.J.
Provincial, Wisconsin Province of the Society of Jesus
February 25, 1999

Library of Congress Cataloging-in-Publication Data

Remembering our home: healing hurts & receiving gifts from conception to birth / by Sheila Fabricant Linn . . . [et al.].
    p.   cm.
Includes bibliographical references.
ISBN 0-8091-3901-4 (alk. paper)
1. Healing—Religious aspects—Christianity. 2. Pregnancy—Religious aspects—Christianity. 3. Psychic trauma—Religious aspects—Christianity.   I. Linn, Sheila Fabricant.
BT732.5.R46   1999
248.8′6—dc21   99-37726
                                                                                CIP

Published by Paulist Press
997 Macarthur Boulevard
Mahwah, New Jersey 07430

www.paulistpress.com

Printed and bound in the United States of America

Table of Contents

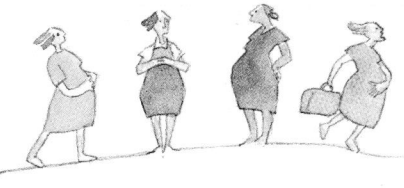

This book is dedicated to

Jamie Emerson-Heery
for allowing me to accompany him
as he finds his way home

and

John Matthew Linn
for helping us remember
the home from which we came.

Our birth is but a sleep and a forgetting:
The Soul that rises with us, our life's Star,
Hath had elsewhere its setting,
And cometh from afar:
Not in entire forgetfulness,
And not in utter nakedness,
But trailing clouds of glory do we come
From God, who is our home:
Heaven lies about us in our infancy!

William Wordsworth
"Ode on Intimations of Immortality"

CHAPTER 1

⚭

Why Should We
Try to Heal Hurts
We Can't Even Remember?

Two years ago, we (Dennis and Sheila) were preparing to adopt a baby. During a long car trip, we listened to audio tapes from a conference on prenatal and perinatal psychology.* The talk that impressed us most was by Dr. William Emerson. For more than thirty years, he has been a pioneer in the treatment of infants and children as well as adults who have experienced prenatal and perinatal trauma. We decided to attend his workshops so that we could learn to be present empathically to the baby who would be ours. We also wanted to resolve any birth traumas that we might have so that we would not pass them on to our child.

At these workshops, we each received profound healing of hurts that went all the way back to conception. We also saw the connection between William's work and our writings and retreats (with Matt) about healing early hurts. For years, the three of us had observed in our ministry of healing prayer what Robin Karr-Morse and Meredith Wiley report in their recent survey of research on early development: "There is no time in human development that equals fetal growth in the speed and complexity—and therefore vulnerability—of development."

As William puts it, prenatal and perinatal hurts tend to form a kind of template or pattern on which later hurts are layered. R.D. Laing agrees:

Prenatal and perinatal psychology means the psychology of babies and their parents during two periods of time: (1) the prenatal period, meaning the time in the womb beginning at conception, and (2) the perinatal period, meaning the time surrounding birth.

The environment is registered from the very beginning of my life, by the very first cell of me. What happens to the first one or two of me may reverberate throughout all subsequent generations of our first cellular parents. That first one of us carries all my genetic memories. . . . It seems to me credible, at least, that all of our experience in our life cycle, from cell one, is absorbed and stored from the beginning—perhaps especially in the beginning. How that may happen I do not know. How can one cell generate the billions and billions of cells I now am? We are impossible except for the fact that we are. When I look at the embryological stages in my . . . life cycle, I experience what feel to me like sympathetic vibrations. How I now feel, I felt then.

Thus, the earliest hurts a person experiences are absorbed and stored in our cells like a remembered tone to which we continue to "vibrate sympathetically." Later hurts then become far more crippling than they otherwise might be. So, for example, a child who was not invited to her classmate's birthday party or a woman whose husband left her would be more devastated by this rejection if her own parents had not wanted to conceive her or had tried to abort her. Similarly, a child who was sent to preschool before he was ready or a man whose home was broken into as an adult would be more devastated by this violation of his sense of security if he was pulled from the womb by cesarean section or by forceps.

We have seen this in our own lives. I (Sheila) was much more devastated by the sexual abuse I experienced as an eight-year-old than I might otherwise have been because my mother was terrified of sexuality at the moment of my conception. I (Dennis) have tended to worry more about being late than I might otherwise because my birth took so long (i.e., I was so late) that I almost died. Our son, John, was especially frightened of male strangers because of the male violence and promiscuity that were so prevalent while he was in his birth mother's womb. We all vibrated sympathetically to the remembered tone of our earliest wounds.

A Paradigm Shift

A paradigm shift is occurring in psychology. This shift is emerging from the realization that prenatal and perinatal wounds have an important and lingering effect on us and that these experiences can have more power over us than experiences in

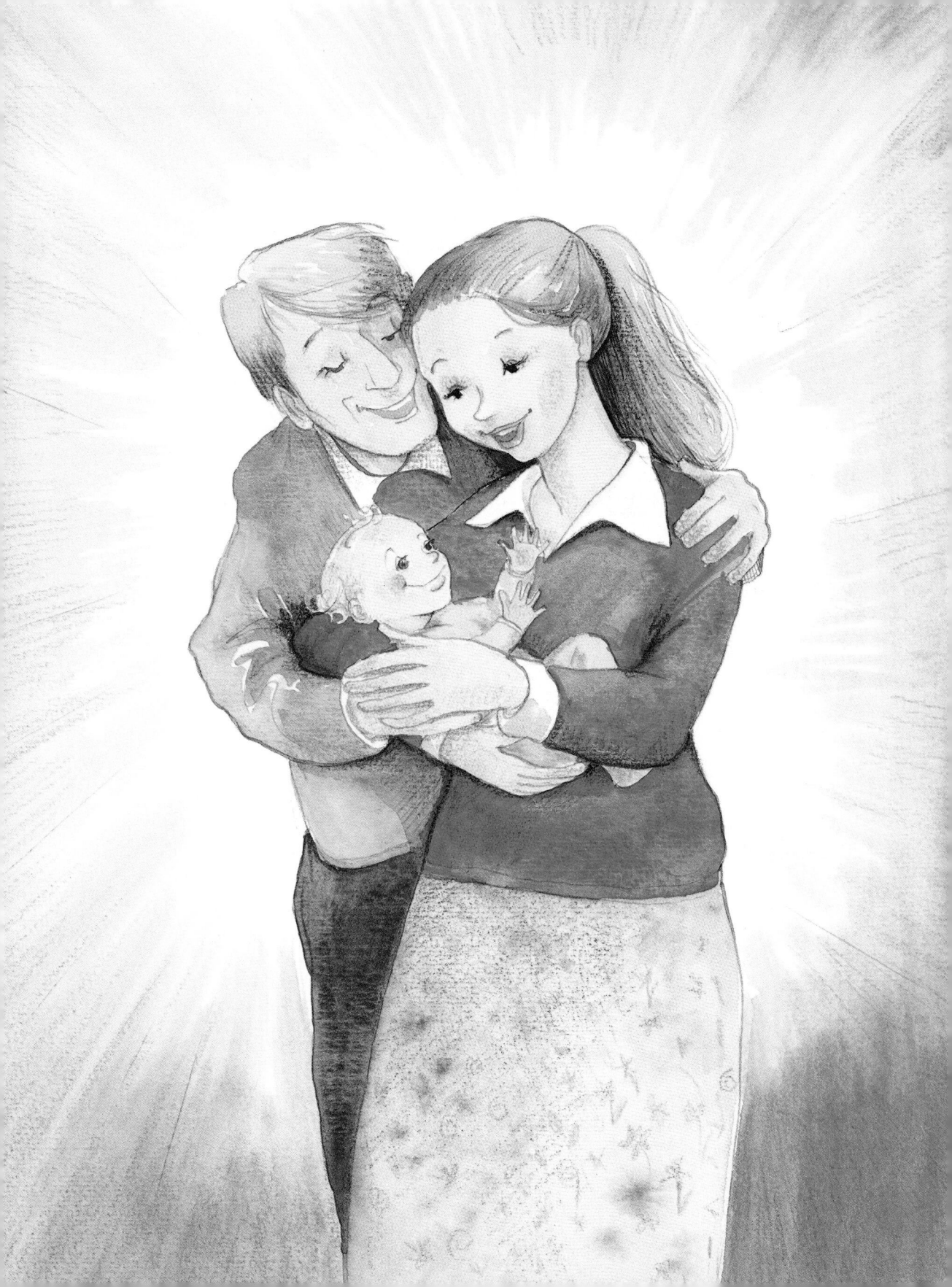

later life. This is a dramatic change from most current thinking. When Freud proposed that early childhood traumas can cause difficulty in adulthood, he initiated a major paradigm shift. Today, Freud's basic insight into the significance of childhood events is generally accepted, and much of psychotherapy is based upon this insight. We believe the work of William and his colleagues represents another major paradigm shift, in which the origin of wounding begins not in childhood but rather at the first moment of our existence. The Western cultural assumption that human beings grow in consciousness as they mature is only half the truth. The opposite is also true: At the moment of conception, a child has a fully conscious spirit that is as sensitive, if not more so, than at any other time in life.

This paradigm shift means not only that we can be wounded earlier than we've thought; it also means we can be healed earlier than we've thought. For example, John has received regular treatment from William, combined with healing prayer, that began when John was three weeks old. He has developed into an extraordinarily healthy, happy, loving, and intelligent child despite the many severe traumas he experienced in the womb and the separation trauma of adoption itself. John will not have to carry prenatal and perinatal wounds into later life, layering hurt upon hurt and using much of his energy to defend himself. He can use his energy to develop his full human potential, and his early wounds can become the basis for a strength of character he might otherwise not achieve. Our experience with John and of the healing of our own prenatal and perinatal trauma have been so profound and so confirming of our ministry that we have now joined William's training program.

William's Story:
How Perinatal Hurts Formed
a Template for My Life

When I (William) was in graduate school preparing to be a psychotherapist, I was required to be in psychotherapy myself. To be a good therapist, I needed to experience the process first. My psychological bias was very traditional. I had been trained in experimental and research psychology, as well as in classical Freudian and Jungian psychology. In my own therapy, I expected to deal with my childhood experiences and perhaps uncover some neurotic patterns, although I considered myself basically normal.

Early in the process, my therapist noted a certain distrust that I had of him and of others and an absence of emotional presence in my work with him. I was surprised because I had always considered myself an emotional and a "feeling" person. Eventually, however, I had to admit that I was quite flat emotionally and not very trusting.

To help me "let go," my therapist suggested that I lie down on his couch and do some deep breathing. During the second or third of these sessions, something very unusual and unexpected happened. I began to shake, sweat, and make sounds. My body felt as if it wanted to roll on its side and push. As I began to push, my feelings escalated and I found myself choking and coughing. I was struggling for my life. Suddenly I realized that I might be experiencing my birth, although at that time (1966) I had never heard of such a thing. The process felt compelling and "right," even though I did not understand it.

As things progressed, I felt as if my twin sister (who died shortly after birth) were right behind me in the birth canal. I reached back, trying to pull her along with me, trying to save her, while trying to birth myself as well. I sensed that we were both at risk of dying and that she might not make it through birth without my help.

During one of the pauses in action, when my feelings subsided somewhat, I heard scurrying and shuffling in the room. I opened my eyes and saw my therapist placing every pillow and couch cushion available around the door in an attempt to prevent sound from escaping. He was disturbed at all the noise I was making and how it might reflect on him. (In those days, sounds were an unusual and unacceptable occurrence when doing psychoanalysis.) Realizing this, I calmed down and began to make my sounds into a pillow, for which my therapist was eternally grateful.

When I told him what I had experienced, he did not believe me. He said that babies could not remember birth, and therefore birth could not have any lasting effect on a child. So I continued to do my birth regressions at home, without him. Intuiting that healing required an environment of empathic love, I found several friends who would compassionately be with me as I regressed. In my regressions I reexperienced the following:

- My mother (and therefore I) was anesthetized. This meant that I lost power in my legs to push and power in my arms to pull my sister, as well as losing my orientation.

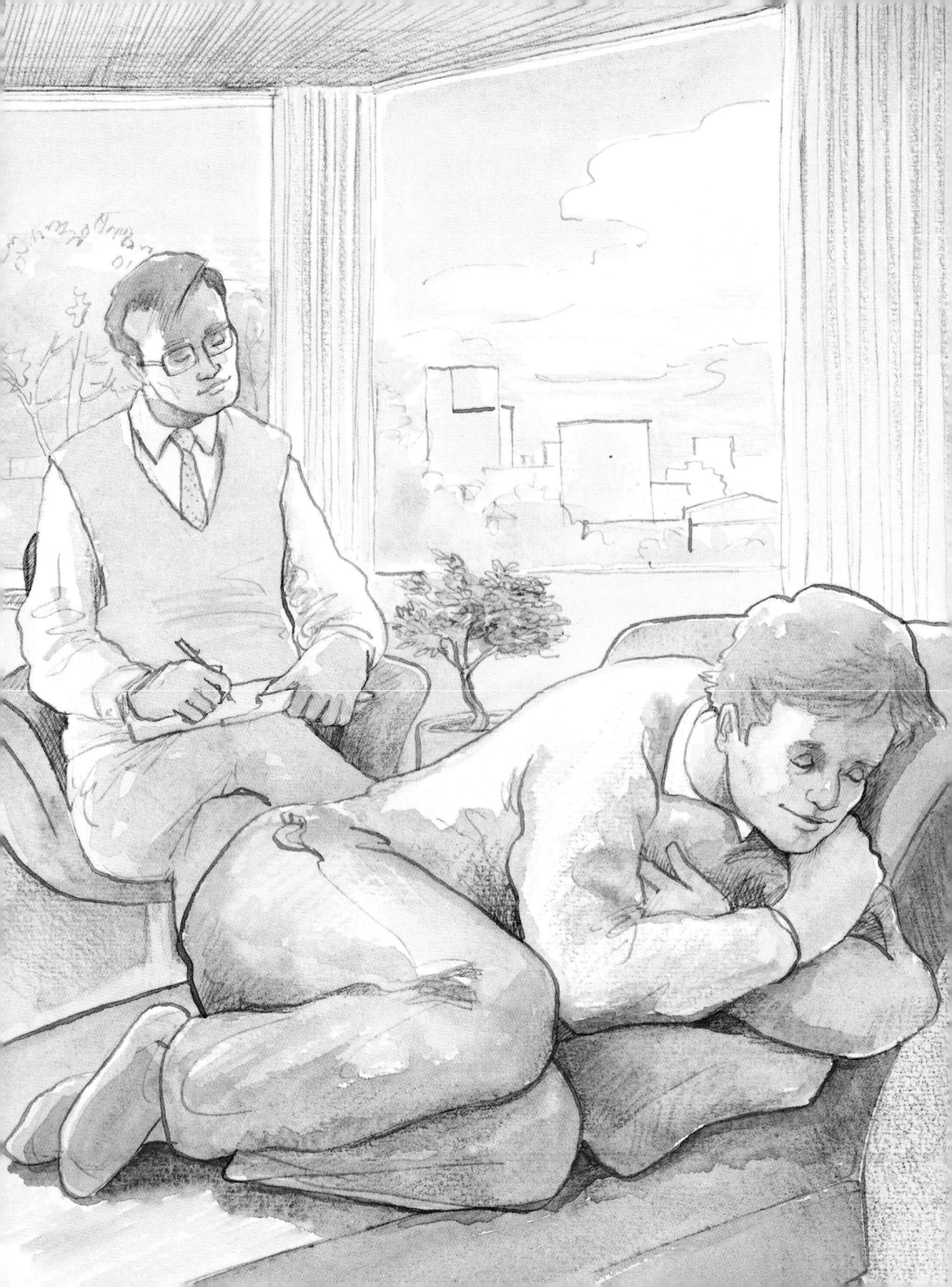

- I was initially breech (feet first) but ultimately born head first.
- My birth weight was extremely low and I was in an incubator for six weeks.
- I was born first, before my sister.
- My sister died twelve hours after birth.
- My mother was depressed after my birth because she had wanted a girl.

When I presented these "facts" to my therapist, he said it would not be possible for me to recall these things. So I went to my birth records. They indicated that I was initially breech, I came first, I was anesthetized, I weighed so little that my chances of survival were virtually·zero, and my twin died twelve hours after birth. My therapist was impressed with the correspondence between my "memories" and my birth records, and he asked if my parents had ever said anything to me about these facts regarding my birth.

So I interviewed my parents (not telling them that I had obtained my birth records). My father, whose memory for life events is excellent, could not recall anything about my birth. My mother said that she thought my birth weight was about three times what I actually did weigh. She didn't recall anesthesia being used. She only remembered that my twin sister had died sometime in the first day after birth. Both of my parents were unaware of any unusual presentation, such as breech. Thus, the story of my birth that I recalled during my regressions, and that matched my hospital records, did not come from my parents.*

What finally compelled me to trust my birth regressions was that I changed so radically afterward. The greatest changes were in my relationships with women, my capacity to be emotionally present to others, and my choice of career.

---

*This is an example of "verification research," in which the birth memories of regressees are compared with objective data such as medical records and/or the memories of those present at the birth, such as parents. Such research has shown birth memories to be highly accurate. In one study in which parents (who had not discussed their children's births with the children) and their children were interviewed separately, their memories of the child's birth were consistent in more than 95% of the cases. In this example, William's memories were not consistent with those of his parents, but it was his *parents* who were mistaken. Especially impressive instances of verification research are those cases in which regressed adults are able to recall, and subsequently confirm, obstetrical interventions despite having been told that such interventions were not used.

I had previously had years of serial relationships with women, in which I felt continually dissatisfied. No woman could ever live up to the intensely harmonious and pleasurable closeness that, in my birth regressions, I recalled having had with my twin sister. Moreover, whenever I was romantically interested in a woman, I would deny my feelings and "sisterize" the relationship, even suggesting to the woman that we call each other "brother" and "sister."

After reexperiencing the loss of my twin during my birth regressions, I grieved her death for several months. I wept a lot during this time, and I am quite sure that my twin would have wept with me if she had been there. Consciously grieving the loss of my twin changed me profoundly. I no longer sisterized my relationships with women. For the first time, I had intimate relationships with hugging and holding that had sexual energy. Now I longed for the woman I was dating, rather than longing for my twin. I didn't fear that women would abandon me, nor did I unconsciously tend to abandon women (which I had done previously as a way to empower myself against abandonment). I've now been happily married for twenty-four years.

Another change that resulted from my birth regressions was that I became a deeply "feeling" person, capable of emotional presence to others. As I began to release my pain and grief, I found an emotional sanctuary within myself where I could experience other feelings as well. In this sanctuary, I found the love of Christ and became able to give it to others by being empathically present to their pain and grief.

The final consequence of my birth regressions was the gift of my career. I had planned to become a traditional Jungian analyst. However, as I got in touch with my own prenatal and perinatal trauma, I was drawn to work with the same hurts in others. I was also drawn toward the compassion of God and its place in regressive work as I came to understand that releasing (or "catharting") primal pain is not, in itself, enough.

I believe that what ultimately heals is an environment of love from others and from God. I learned this during the time when I was connecting with the deep despair and sadness I carried from my prenatal and perinatal wounding. As I released my emotions through crying, shaking, and wailing, a profound healing occurred. However, one aspect of my wounding did not change: My feelings of aloneness and alienation were still present and active, both in my regressions and in my life. One evening, as I began to cry and wail, I finally and spontaneously called out to God, "Please help me." I immediately felt God's presence and understanding.

God said to me, "Of course I know you, of course I feel your pain, and of course I am with you." I knew God's immense compassion for me. I realized that my screams, my cries, and my despair had been heard by God, and I experienced a significant shift that was an essential part of my healing.

Thus, my profound early wounding became my doorway to God. The wounds that occur when we're very young—particularly the wounds that occur before language develops—are stored in the crevices and subtle areas of the inner self where our instinctual life begins. We are created in the image of God, as we are told in Genesis 1:27, and the presence of God permeates those same deep spaces in the inner self. Therefore, when we access and heal our deepest wounds, we also access the deepest spaces within us where God dwells.

Matt's Story:
How Prenatal Hurts
Formed a Template for My Life

I (Matt) was so moved to hear of Dennis and Sheila's experience with William that I, too, joined his training program. During a regression process, with the help of guided imagery accompanied by deep breathing, I reexperienced my prenatal life. I felt helpless and defenseless, as if I were in the middle of a war. I saw boats sinking, bombs falling, and fire everywhere. I felt my father's fear of being taken from his home and forced into a violent conflict in a faraway place. I felt my mother's fear that something really terrible could go wrong. I wanted to make it right. I made an inner vow to fix whatever I could, believing that things could always get worse, perhaps even threatening my very survival.

During the regression, I prayed for an image that would embody and heal all this fear. I saw myself struggling to stay alive in the face of a firestorm. But my fear remained until I imagined myself being killed and swept into God's hands forever. I didn't have to survive! I could die and be safe in God.

In the days following this regression, I began to understand its meaning. I was born during World War II. My parents' safe world was destroyed by the bombing of Pearl Harbor on December 7, l941, which was the start of the draft my father feared. Her fear of losing her husband and raising a child alone was a daily reality for my pregnant mother. I researched the newspapers that my parents were reading during

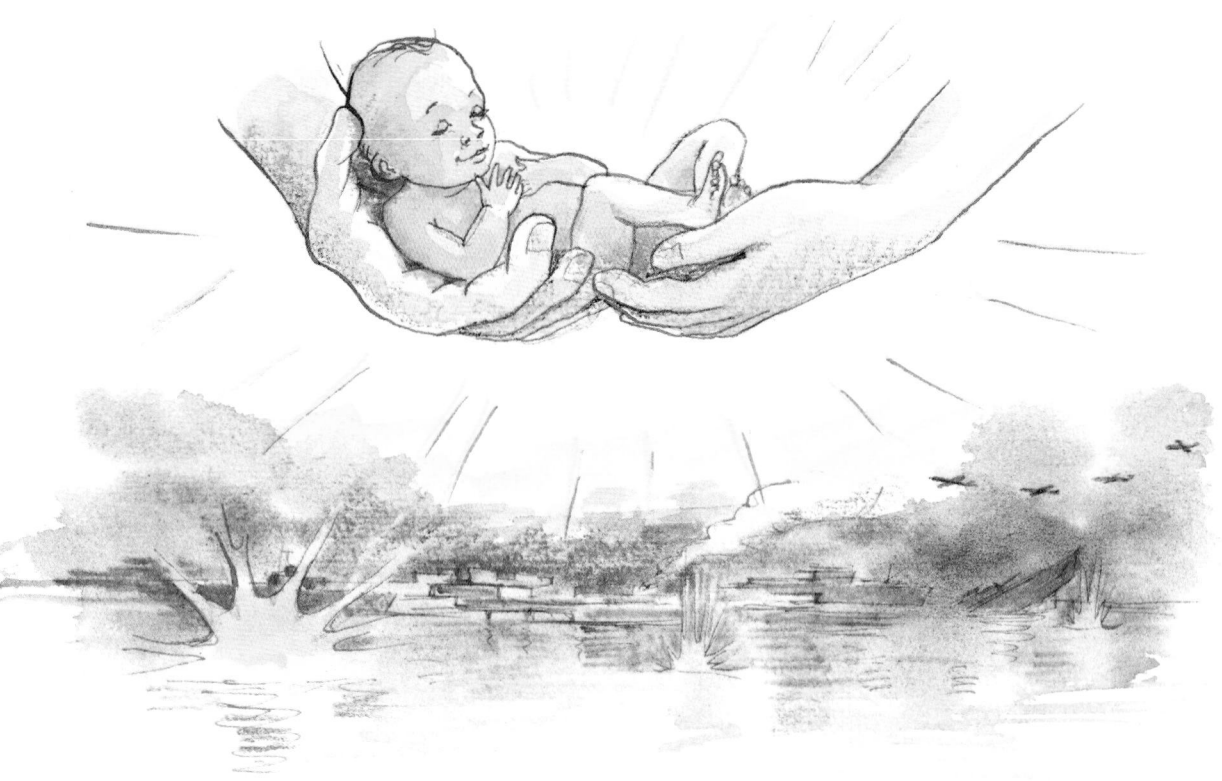

the nine months prior to my birth in October 1942, and I found fear and defeat on every page—the same fear that has dominated my life.

My personality has always been dominated by fear in the form of a desire to fix things and solve problems. My ministry is devoted to giving retreats and writing books with Dennis and Sheila on how people can solve their problems. However, I tend to overuse this gift. For example, when visiting Dennis and Sheila, I used to pull up every weed in their yard. Then I would go next door and pull up the *neighbor's* weeds! As a spiritual director, I would give unsolicited advice before I even understood the problem.

Since the regression, I have noticed that I no longer feel compelled to pull up weeds but do it only when I want to exercise. (And I haven't even touched the weeds in the neighbor's yard.) My desk has a growing pile of unfinished business and unsolved problems that I could never have tolerated before. I have also noticed that now I would rather spend time playing with Dennis and Sheila's baby, John Matthew, than fixing things. Perhaps by coming to peace with my inner prenate (the unborn child I once was and still carry within me), I am more at peace with John's infantile behavior. When he empties the cupboards, he helps heal me of my need to have things all fixed up. After I've cleaned up three times and then watched John throw everything back on the floor, I am able to adopt his view of the world. John's world is in order when the floor is covered with things to explore . . . which looks like chaos and disorder to me. When I still find that I compulsively want to fix the disorder around me, I return to my prenatal memory and the image of being protected in God's arms.

We Recapitulate Unhealed Hurts

Matt's story is an example of how, when an early hurt is unresolved, an adult may continually create situations that reenact the original hurt and/or that completely avoid its recurrence. This process, known as recapitulation, is how we (unconsciously) keep reminding ourselves of the template, or the "familiar tone to which we continue to vibrate sympathetically." Thus, Matt recapitulated his prenatal experience by seeking out problems to fix and even created problems where there were none so that World War II would still be going on around him. This is known as direct recapitulation. If, on the other hand, Matt went to the opposite extreme and avoided problems that required solving or fixing, then his pattern would be characteristic of avoidant recapitulation.

How Can We Experience Our Parents' World While We Are in the Womb?

How could Matt have experienced his parents' fear while he was in the womb, to the extent that later he continually recapitulated fears related to World War II in his everyday life? At one level, Matt could have experienced his parents' world through his biological connection to his mother. Every emotion a pregnant woman feels produces chemical changes in her blood; these changes are then shared with her child as they cross the placenta and enter the child's body through the umbilical cord. Just how quickly mother and child can share feelings is demonstrated by an experiment in which pregnant women were told that their babies weren't moving. Each woman became alarmed that something might be wrong with her baby. Within seconds, the baby, observed through ultrasound, was kicking—apparently in response to his or her mother's fear.

At a more subtle and mysterious level, babies have a spiritual connection to their parents and to their parents' world. Perhaps you can understand this by recalling moments when you have thought of a friend who was far away and at that very moment received a phone call from that person, or you may have experienced entering a room and feeling uneasy, only to learn that a terrible argument had just taken place there.

Clinical researchers have observed that babies, too, have a kind of intuitive radar that allows them to pick up feelings and subtle changes in their environment. Perhaps this is how Matt picked up his father's fear of being drafted and even pictured scenes of things taking place in Europe that his parents were not directly experiencing. Babies marinate in the mental, emotional, and spiritual climate of their parents' inner lives, and their consciousness is permeated by their parents' world. Thus, prenatal and perinatal trauma includes not only those events we experienced directly, but also ways in which we were permeated by our parents' unresolved trauma and the trauma of the world in which they lived.

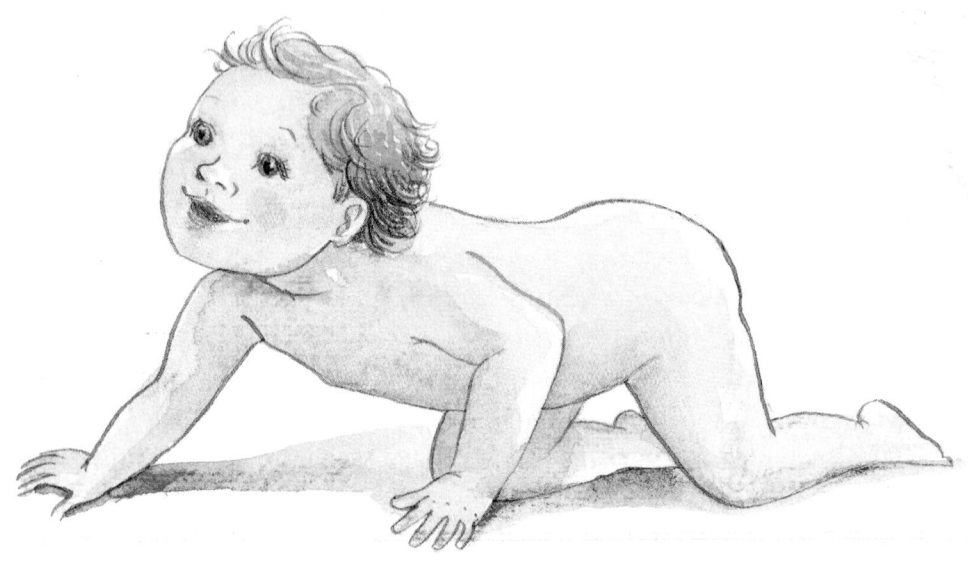

Beginning at the Beginning

Unresolved prenatal and perinatal trauma can have devastating long-term effects not only on the individual but also on society. Several years ago, the state of California funded the first scientific study of the roots of violence and crime. The study concluded that a significant factor in the increase of violence in our culture is the separation of mother and infant at birth.

Why is the separation of mother and infant at birth predictive of violence? Erik Erikson identified the task of the first stage of life, infancy, as the formation of basic trust. If basic trust is not achieved, all later stages of development into a moral, loving, and responsible adult are compromised. The "stuff" of trust in infancy is bonding, meaning a mutual process of attachment in which the adult experiences commitment to the baby and the baby experiences trust of the adult. When a baby is separated from his or her mother at birth—the moment he or she is most ready to begin the bonding process outside the womb—the baby's capacity to trust is deeply wounded. In our culture, other assaults on trust often follow. They include things we regard as normal, such as circumcision, invasive medical procedures, insufficient breast-feeding, requiring infants to sleep alone in cribs, and putting babies in day care after a standard six-week maternity leave. In addition, the language of babies, their crying, is often suppressed. Babies communicate their feelings through crying, and for healthy bonding to occur, these feelings need to be listened to.

Moreover, as William's work emphasizes, disruption in bonding can begin long before the separation of mother and child at birth. It can begin as early as conception, through such things as ambivalence about the pregnancy, conflict or anger between the parents, substance abuse, and sexuality that involves power, force, or violence. All of these contribute to the current epidemic of violence among our adolescents and adults. We also see symptoms of disrupted bonding in the pervasive cynicism, materialism (attachment to things rather than to persons), and emphasis on self-interest throughout our society. Well-bonded human beings who have developed basic trust do not behave in these ways.

In an effort to address these problems, many concerned people in the United States have promoted Head Start (a program of intellectual and social enrichment for deprived preschool-age children). More recently, Early Head Start was designed to focus on even younger children, from ages zero to three. In Venezuela, from 1979 to 1984, the government promoted Project Family. Like Early Head Start, it was designed to stimulate the full development of children from poor families, beginning at birth. However, in comparison with their peers, the gains made by the children in Project Family were only temporary.

The director of Project Family, Dr. Beatriz Manrique, realized that to have a lasting impact, she needed to begin earlier, in the womb. She designed an enrichment program called Hello Baby, that began during the fifth month of gestation and continued until age six. The follow-up study of these children is the largest experimental study of prenatal enrichment to date. It shows that they made lasting physical, emotional, intellectual, and social gains. Hello Baby demonstrates that programs like Head Start—even Early Head Start—are too late. If we really want to help our children, ourselves, and our culture, we have to begin at the beginning.

We Came from the Heart of God

The beginning was good. Although some of us may no longer remember, we all came from the heart of God. This is our true home. In this home, God, as with Jeremiah, knew us intimately before we were even in the womb:

> The word of Yahweh was addressed to me, saying, "Before I formed you in the womb I knew you, before you came to birth I consecrated you; I have appointed you as prophet to the nations." (Jer 1:4–5)

The Hebrew word that we translate as "knew" is *yada*, which does not refer to vague knowledge but rather to the deepest possible intimacy, in which one knows the most hidden part of a person. For example, *yada* is commonly used to refer to sexual intercourse (as in Gn 4:1). Thus, before we were formed in the womb, God knew every part of us.

We (Dennis, Sheila, and Matt) suggested calling this book *Remembering Our Home* because the greatest effect on us of our work with William has been to help us remember where we came from. An image for this is the experience that the three of us have often had with dying people. As we accompany such people, we seem to glimpse the doorway ahead of them through which they will pass from this world into the heart of God. Similarly, in our work with birth trauma, we have glimpsed the doorway behind us through which we passed into this world from our home in the heart of God.

We want to receive from John his memory of the heart of God. Up until around age five, many children report memories of their life with God before birth. We've come to believe that the main task of parents (and uncles and everyone else who cares about them) is to help children preserve their memory of having come from the heart of God. We might also say that the main task of spouses, friends, therapists, pastoral workers, and so on is to help those with whom they relate to remember that they, too, came from the heart of God.

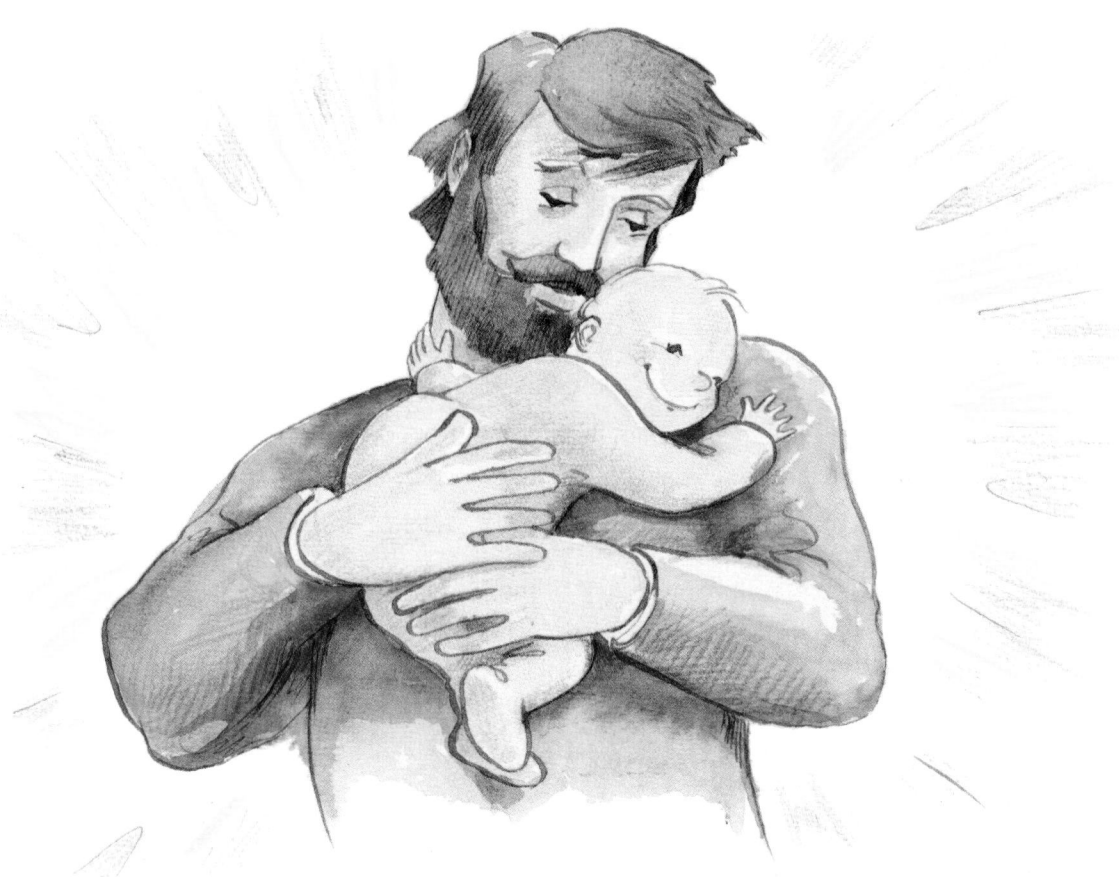

Mapping the Beginning of Life

Our ministry is based on the integration of spirituality with recent developments in psychology and medicine. In this book, we will integrate spirituality with what we have learned from William about healing prenatal and perinatal hurts. In the field of prenatal and perinatal psychology, William is regarded as a courageous pioneer. For thirty years, he conducted clinical research with his infant, child, and adult clients. He did regression therapy, took extensive notes, and did thorough follow-up evaluations with all his clients. It is they who taught William the map of prenatal life and its impacts on later life that he will share in the chapters that follow.

Perhaps William's "mapping" of the experience of babies in the womb can be compared to the work of another pioneer, Raymond Moody, who first mapped near-death experiences (NDEs) in the 1970s. Although many people had shared NDEs with him, these experiences were initially met with skepticism by the scientific community. Now, however, Moody's map of NDEs is generally accepted as a universal and valid human experience. Similarly, although William's work may seem "stretching" to some of our readers, it is grounded in embryological research as well as anecdotal reports from thousands of his clients (an anecdotal report is a client's account of his or her personal experience).

Dr. David Chamberlain, a highly respected clinical and research psychologist, says that anecdotal data

> . . . are especially precious because they are human experiences, pointing the way for fruitful exploration, and warning us of realities ten or twenty years before any confirmation we can hope to get from formal experiments.

We believe that in ten or twenty years, William's insights into the beginning of life may become as widely accepted as Moody's insights into the end of life.

Final Words of Welcome to the Reader

I (William) am happy to collaborate with Dennis, Sheila, and Matt in integrating prenatal and perinatal psychology with methods of healing prayer. I am also eager to make the healing of early trauma as widely available as possible.

This book is not intended as a substitute for psychotherapy. If you have problems that require professional treatment, you should seek help from trained medical and/or psychological professionals. If, as you do any of the exercises suggested in this book, you experience troubling symptoms, you should stop the exercise and likewise seek professional help.

Although we (Dennis, Sheila, and Matt) write as Christians in the Roman Catholic tradition, we hope our inclusion of experiences that are universal will make this book equally healing for people of other religious traditions. As many studies collected by physician Dr. Larry Dossey demonstrate, the power of prayer is not determined by the religious tradition of the one who prays. Dr. Dossey writes,

> As long as love, empathy and compassion are present, the prayer seems to work. . . . I feel there is a great lesson in tolerance in these experiments in prayer. When it comes to prayer, no religion has a monopoly.

Whatever your religious tradition, our hope is that you can translate anything we've written into a form that will be healing and life-giving for you and your children.

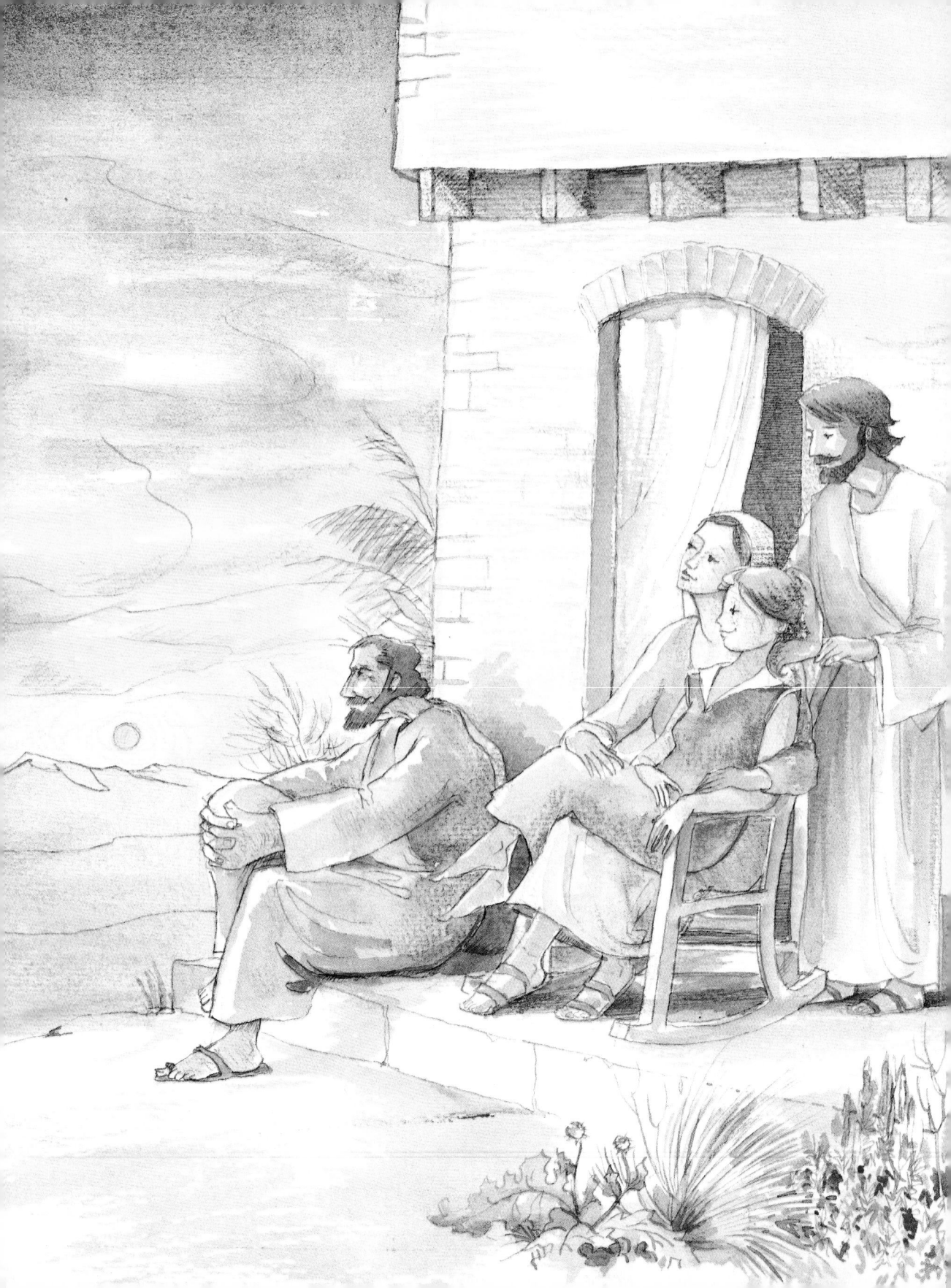

CHAPTER 2

❧

Healing of Prenatal and Perinatal Trauma Is for Everyone

Although much of what we (Dennis, Sheila, and Matt) have learned from William is new to us, we (and our colleagues in ministry) have seen many people healed when, in prayer, they spontaneously regressed to birth, the womb, or even conception. They have shared with us how Jesus, Mary, or another trusted figure entered the scene and helped them.

Healing by Inviting Jesus to Enter Our Life

I (Sheila) experienced this at my first workshop with William. As William led us in a guided meditation to regress to our births, I felt terror and grief at the realization that I would have to leave the womb. Although my birth was very difficult physically, that was not my primary concern. Rather, I was aware that I was being born to mentally ill parents who would not be able to *see* me—really see me as myself. I could remember the heart of God behind me. I knew that I had been seen there, and I felt great despair at losing that.

In this guided meditation, I asked God for help, and an image came to me that has recurred often in my prayer. The image is of a small, ancient house in the old city of Jerusalem, overlooking a valley to the west. In the doorway, there is a rocking chair. Although Jesus did not live in Jerusalem as far as we know, I imagine him there, at home with his family. One or another of them holds me and rocks me in the chair.

As I look out, I see the sun setting. The brilliant color across the sky represents to me the immense creative power of God, and the one who holds me represents the intimate personal love of God. The chair in the doorway is the intersection of the two—the intersection of heaven and earth, of God's transcendence and God's immanence. In that chair, I always have the sense that I am rocking across eternity.

As I rocked in the chair in my imagination during the regression process, I realized that the same eternal depth of being—the image of God—was within me. The scene that surrounded me in the doorway of Jesus' home was a mirror of my spirit. I felt even more deeply my longing to be seen at birth, in all my depth and as clearly as the one who held me in the chair could see me. Then I realized that I came here knowing that eventually I would meet Denny and he would see me. With that, I felt willing to be born. It occurred to me that Jesus' family would go with me as I left the womb and that I could simply rock my way out. So that's what I imagined myself doing. It was easy and joyful. Denny, who was my partner in the regression process, welcomed me and communicated his delight in my birth.

Since then, a memory of my home in the heart of God that I have had all my life has become much more vivid and central to my awareness. I feel a new conviction that the loving light from which I came will never leave me and that I am *seen* as I live out my life here. Moreover, it's all right to *be* seen. Although I often speak to large groups and am usually quite comfortable, before this process I felt extreme shyness and self-consciousness in any group in which I was not the speaker. Now, I am increasingly comfortable being seen by others, even when I do not have the protection of the special role of speaker.

Because this birth regression experience was so healing for me, I returned to it often as I became a mother. During the first months of John's life, I often worried that I would not be a good enough mother because I did not receive good mothering myself. I recalled a story by the psychiatrist, Robert Coles. During the Civil Rights movement, he interviewed the families of African American children in the South who were involved in integrating the schools. One six-year-old child had marched through crowds of people who yelled at her, threw things at her, and turned water hoses on her. The child lived in an extended family that included her grandmother. Robert Coles asked her mother, "How can you endure this?" The mother said, "*My mother puts her hands on me, and I put my hands on my child.*"

I knew that I needed someone to put their hands on me to help me put my hands on my child. So, since John came, I often see myself in that rocking chair in the doorway of the house in Jerusalem. I imagine Jesus' family behind me, putting their hands on my back. Then I ask God to help me put my hands on my son in the same loving way.

Healing by Going to Be with Jesus in His Life

In healing prayer, we invite Jesus (or some other trusted person) into any painful moment in our lives and receive *now* the healing love that we needed *then*. This is possible because there is no chronological time in God. What Sheila has just described is one form of healing prayer, in which we get in touch with a scene from our own life and ask Jesus to enter that scene and help us. Another form of healing prayer is going to be with Jesus (or another person who mediates God's healing love) in a scene from his life. So, instead of asking Jesus to come to be with us, we go to be with him.

For example, I (Dennis) grew up with a fear of women and of sexuality. I never dated in high school, and for the next twenty-seven years, I lived in a celibate religious community. As usually happens when something healthy is repressed, my sexuality came out in compulsive and unhealthy ways. After I learned about healing prayer, I asked myself what I wanted from Jesus' life. I realized that I wanted to go to Bethlehem and be held by Mary, as Jesus was. So I imagined myself in the stable at Bethlehem being held by Mary and even being breast-fed by her. I did this every day for two or three months until the desire for it was gone. During the next several months, I noticed that my fear of women gradually disappeared. My compulsive sexual behaviors also ceased. I formed healthy friendships with women and experienced a new sense of wholeness in my sexual identity. It is a miracle to me that now I am happily married to Sheila.

I could have spent years trying to figure out where my fear of women came from and why I struggled with sexuality. Often, such introspection, perhaps with the help of a therapist and/or a spiritual companion, would be very valuable for personal growth. However, sometimes healing comes simply by asking for it. In this case, I asked Jesus for what I most wanted from his life—to be held by his mother. What I most wanted was what I most needed for healing, without having to figure it out in my head.

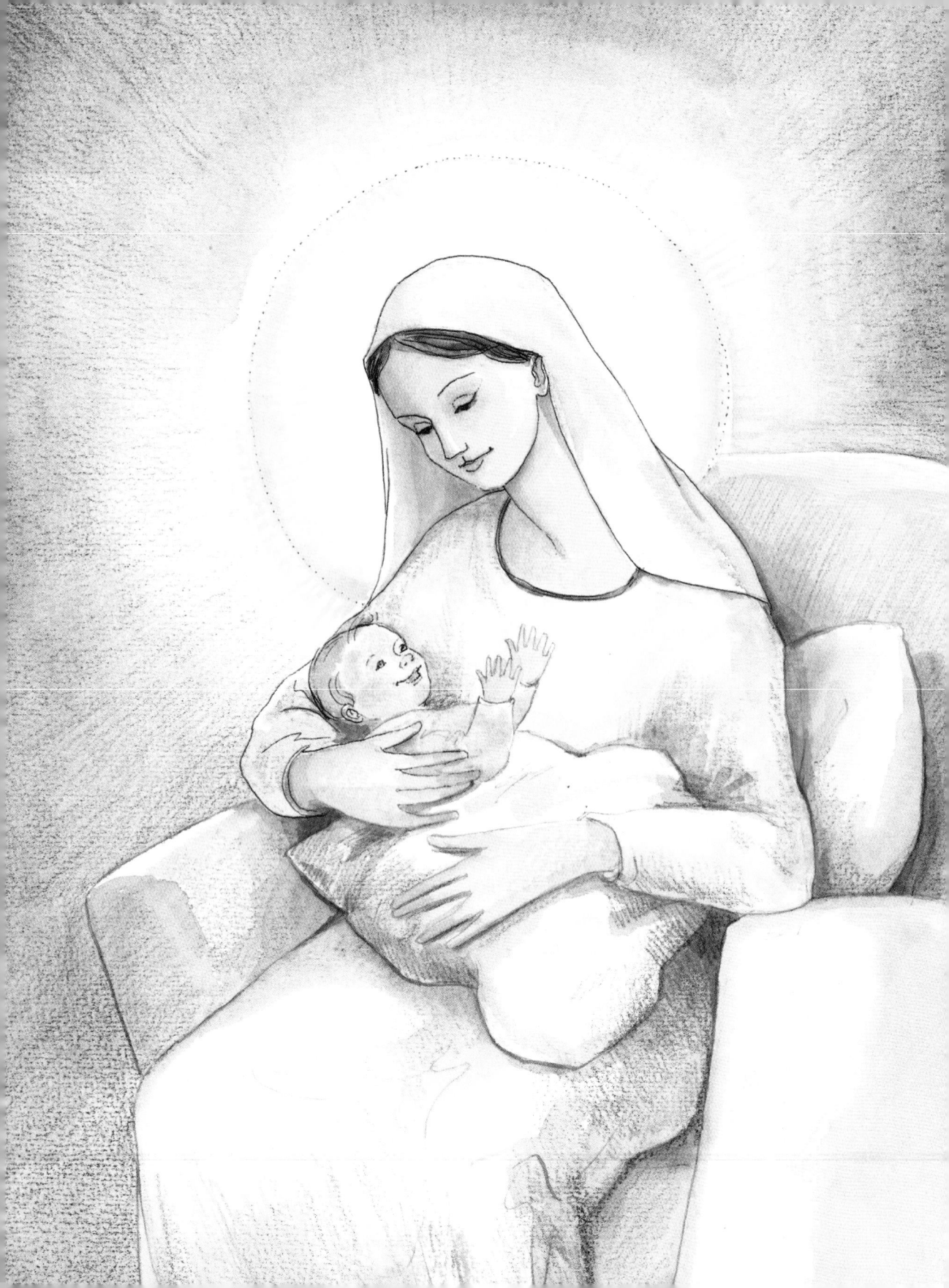

Healing and Religious Imagery

In the above examples of healing prayer, Dennis and Sheila each drew upon images from scripture. We believe that praying in this way is healing for at least three reasons. First, as mentioned earlier, Jesus and his family are real presences who are actively capable of communicating healing love to us, simply because we need it. This is healing through divine intervention.

Second, imagination is a powerful source of healing. When we imaginatively join Jesus in a scene from his life or ask him to join us in a scene from our life, we are evoking the power of our imagination in a context of love.

Third, biblical imagery is exquisitely and mysteriously designed to evoke the depths of our own inner life. The archetypal symbols of the Bible—rich as they are in prenatal and perinatal themes such as journeys, discoveries, and homes—can activate our own wounds that are ready for healing, including those of which we were unaware. We say "are ready for healing," because we trust that in an environment of love (rather than one of insensitive probing), generally only those traumas that are ready for healing will emerge into consciousness.

When I (Sheila) went to be with the Holy Family in their home in Jerusalem, their love for one another expanded my capacity to imagine a loving home. It also put me more deeply in touch with the trauma of my birth and the depth of my longing for a safe family to welcome me. At the same time, I experienced the Holy Family as a resource to meet my longing.

When I (Dennis) went to be held by Mary, her warmth expanded my capacity to imagine even being breast-fed by her. It also put me in touch with the trauma of not being breast-fed by my own mother, a trauma of which I was not previously aware. At the same time, I experienced Mary as one who could heal me.

Our experience with healing prayer is confirmed by studies of the use of religious imagery. For example, in a study by psychologist L.R. Propst of depressed patients who scored high on measures of religiosity, some received therapy that encouraged religious imagery, and others received the same therapy but without the use of religious imagery. Only 14 percent of the patients in the first group remained depressed, compared to 60 percent of the patients in the second group, whose therapy did not include religious imagery.

Because religious imagery is so powerful and has been so healing of my own early trauma, I imagine our son, John, in Mary's womb so that he can receive from

Mary all that he did not receive in his birth mother's womb. I especially do this each evening when Sheila and I pin a medal of Our Lady of Guadalupe to his pajamas. The medal is a reminder of the many times we have visited the Shrine of Our Lady of Guadalupe in Mexico City. Perhaps one reason why so much healing has happened there is that Our Lady of Guadalupe wears a sash to indicate that she is pregnant. Maybe the Mexican people and pilgrims from all over the world love her so much and keep returning to visit her because they have found a way to heal prenatal and perinatal trauma by relating to her. Thus, I expect that bringing John to Mary's womb is healing him, especially as he sleeps, just as her breast-feeding healed me and just as her presence at the Shrine of Our Lady of Guadalupe has healed so many pilgrims.

The Spiritual Exercises

When I went to be with Jesus in a scene from his life and allowed Mary to breast-feed me, I did what St. Ignatius recommends in the *Spiritual Exercises*. St. Ignatius was the founder of the Jesuit religious order to which I belonged. His retreat manual, the *Spiritual Exercises*, is used as the basis for many retreats in the Catholic tradition. One common aspect of these spiritual exercises is to imagine oneself participating with Jesus in the events of his life as recorded in the gospels.

The retreatant joins Jesus in his conception and continues through Jesus' gestation, birth, childhood, and the events of his life up through his death and resurrection. The retreatant is encouraged to enter a given scene, identify with Jesus, and take in from Jesus whatever he or she needs for healing. The assumption here is that Jesus is, today, a real and living presence who wants to and can give us everything he has.

Healing Is for Everyone

This kind of healing process is one that we do consciously, because it is our life's work. We have given hundreds of retreats in which we've led hundreds of thousands of people in entering a scene like Jesus' birth at Bethlehem. Some of the therapists who have attended our retreats keep a crib scene in their office and often invite their clients to go to Bethlehem to receive healing.

But what about people who never come to a retreat, never go to a therapist, and never attend a workshop with someone like William? Those of us who participate in Christian culture are, nevertheless, exposed to opportunities for healing prenatal and perinatal trauma. For example, our culture's favorite Christian feast is Christmas. Many of our Christmas traditions are ways of healing our prenatal and perinatal trauma by imaginatively participating in Jesus' conception, gestation, and birth.

The crib scene, introduced by St. Francis of Assisi, is an especially popular way of preparing for Christmas. Francis took a donkey and an ox into a cave in the forest. Then he used wood and straw to build a manger there, with a carved wooden figure of the baby Jesus. Local villagers played the parts of Joseph, Mary, and the shepherds. Hundreds of people came to see the crib scene, and the night sky was lit up by their torches.

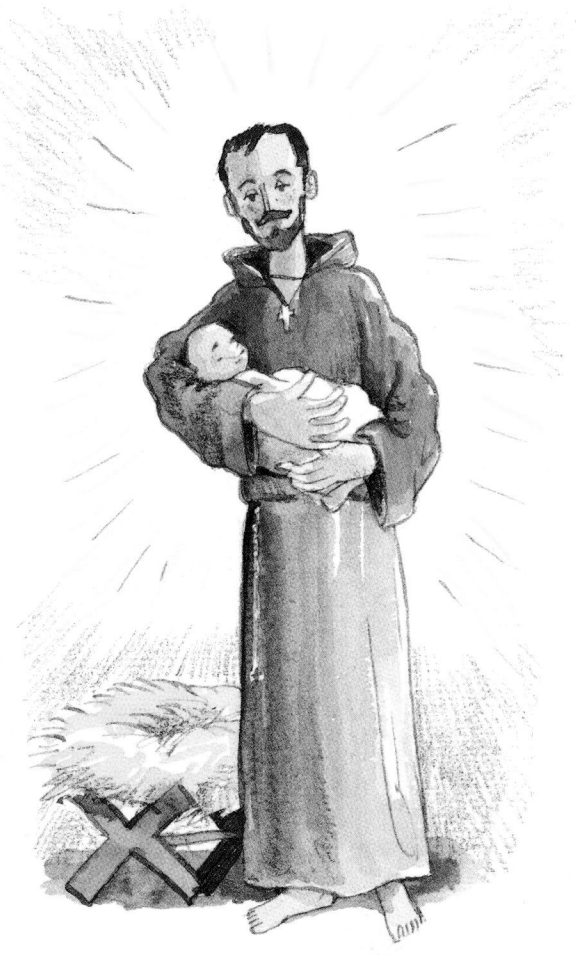

A knight who was present, John of Greccio, claimed that, instead of a wooden figure, he saw a beautiful child asleep in the manger crib and that St. Francis took him in his arms and the child woke up. Our guess is that John of Greccio's own inner child realized his beauty and woke up. We don't know that, but we do know that the people kept the hay from the crib as a reminder of what they experienced that night. The hay was said to heal their illnesses as well as to cure their animals.

As children, all during Advent after Sunday Mass, our (Dennis and Matt's) family would stand in line waiting our turn to place straw carefully in the church manger. The manger was empty (the child Jesus would be placed there on Christmas Eve). In this way, the entire church congregation participated in Jesus' gestation and birth. Our eighty-seven-year-old mother still attends that church, and this year we will again stand in line with her, waiting to place our straw carefully in the manger.

The crib scene has become a symbol for the whole Christian world of participation in Jesus' birth, rather like a collective projective technique. We are instinctively doing what St. Ignatius recommended by entering a scene from Jesus' life. We each do this in our own way. For example, two years ago, we found the most extensive crib scene we've ever seen in a church in Oaxaca, Mexico. Oaxaca is one of Mexico's major centers for raising sheep. We've never seen a crib scene with so many sheep—there were hundreds of them. Also, the people had located the crib scene not in Bethlehem but in the midst of the rolling hills of Oaxaca. Around the stable in which Jesus was born were miniature versions of the people's homes as well as other images typical of the daily life of the people of Oaxaca, such as women pounding corn. It looked as if every family might have brought something to add to the scene. Thus, they were symbolically integrating their own lives with the birth of Jesus.

Another example is the crib scene given us (Dennis and Sheila) by our nephew, David. He made it for us as a wedding gift, when he was seven years old. In that crib

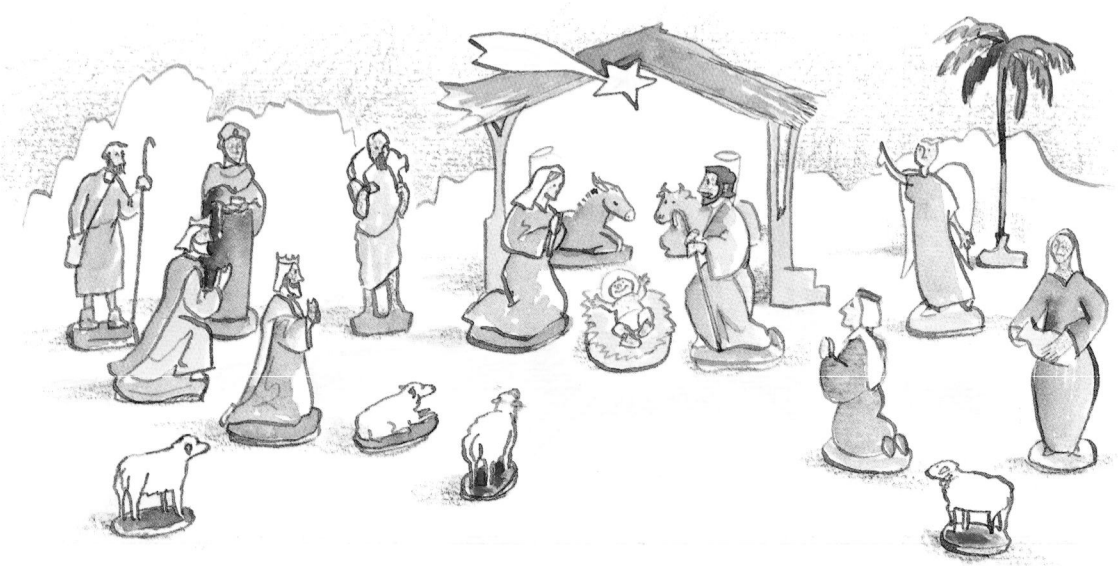

scene, Jesus' mother looks like David's mother, Mary Ellen. She even has the same pouffy hairdo. There are no sheep; in fact, David painted over the one image of a sheep that was embossed on the back wall of the stable. Maybe David's lack of interest in sheep comes from the fact that David's parents own several Burger King restaurants. If a cow had been embossed in the back wall of the cave, it probably would have survived!

What David did is what the Italian and French painters did as well. They painted the nativity scenes full of people who looked like their own families or the royal family that sponsored their painting. Perhaps they, too, were identifying with the life of Jesus to open their unconscious in order to receive healing from the crib scene. From our point of view, this isn't just a projective technique—although it is that—but a way of actually accessing the healing love of God and letting it touch and heal our prenatal and perinatal wounds.

Although we doubt that St. Ignatius ever heard the words *projective technique*, he seems to have intuitively understood the need to integrate one's own experience imaginatively with Jesus' birth in a way that could bring healing. Even though Ignatius visited Jesus' birthplace and remembered it in detail, he encouraged retreatants to create their own pictures of the place where Jesus was born. For example, he writes that one should "Observe the place or cave where Christ is born; whether big or little; whether high or low; and how it is arranged." Ignatius's words seem to us a medieval form of the meditations by which William has helped us reexperience the womb and the birth tunnel from which we came, "whether big or little, high or low" and whether its arrangement includes many obstacles.

Healing Prenatal and Perinatal Trauma in the Gospels

When Ignatius invites us to reconstruct scenes from Jesus' prenatal and perinatal life imaginatively in ways that most fit our needs for healing, he is imitating the gospels. The account of Jesus' birth occurs in the Gospels of Matthew and Luke, and his birthplace is referred to in the Gospels of John and Mark as well as elsewhere in the New Testament. Because the audiences of the gospel writers were as different from one another as the royal audiences of the French and Italian painters were from the shepherds of Oaxaca, the birth stories of each writer are very different. The events before, during, and after Jesus' birth are reported so differently that it seems to many prominent scholars (such as Raymond Brown and John Meier) that no one person could do them all. For example:

- How could Jesus be born in both Bethlehem, as the Infancy Narratives in Luke and Matthew suggest, and at the same time be born in Nazareth as the entire rest of the New Testament assumes, including the Gospels of John (1:45, 7:41–42) and Mark (6:1–4)?*
- How could Jesus be born in Joseph's home in Bethlehem, as Matthew suggests, and at the same time be born in an abandoned stable far away from home as Luke suggests?
- In Matthew's gospel, the celebration of Jesus' birth is cut short by the narrow escape of Jesus into Egypt to avoid King Herod's slaughter of Jewish babies. In Luke's gospel, the celebration of Jesus' birth continues. There is no King Herod, no slaughter of Jewish babies, no flight into Egypt. Instead, Jesus returns home to Nazareth after his birth.

These discrepancies have led many scholars to conclude that the gospel writers were not writing biographical history, but rather symbolic history based on images from the Old Testament to affirm that Jesus is Savior. We wonder if they were also, perhaps unconsciously, trying to heal their own prenatal and perinatal hurts and those of their readers. Perhaps they told the story differently because their audiences were different and they were creating a safe and familiar environment in which hurts could be healed.

I (Sheila) did exactly the same thing with that scene of the rocking chair in the ancient house in Jerusalem. I imagine this as the place where Jesus was born and raised, even though most scholars would probably agree that Jesus was born and lived in Nazareth. However, Jerusalem is extremely significant for *me*. Each time I've

---

*Raymond Brown writes that apart from the Infancy Narratives in Matthew and Luke, "there is not only a silence in the rest of the NT about Bethlehem as the birthplace of Jesus; there is positive evidence for Nazareth and Galilee as Jesus' hometown or native region: his *patris*." Brown says, for example, that *patris* in Mark 6:1–4 refers to Nazareth and means "birthplace."

been there, I have felt especially close to my Jewish ancestors who can put their hands on me in ways that my mother could not. Thus, I'm integrating a symbol of strength and comfort in my own life (Jerusalem) with my experience of Jesus and his family as sources of love. I'm imaginatively creating a safe place, a "holding environment," an inner "eternal city" in which I can receive healing.

Not only Christmas but other feasts are also times for healing. One is the Annunciation, which we celebrate on March 25, nine months before Jesus' birth. This feast celebrates how an angel announced to Mary that she would conceive Jesus and how Mary said "Yes." The Annunciation reminds us that each of us needs to be chosen even before we are conceived. It can also activate our own memories surrounding conception.

Another feast related to Jesus' birth is the Visitation, on May 31. The Visitation celebrates how, early in her pregnancy, Jesus' mother visited her pregnant cousin, Elizabeth. It can activate our own memories of how we were welcomed or not welcomed by others as we were carried in our mother's womb. The Visitation also celebrates the conscious life of the child in the womb as the two babies (Jesus and John the Baptist) communicate with each other and become lifelong friends.

Healing and the Imagination

Some of the healing processes we will suggest are based on the Christian feasts we have mentioned. All the healing processes are simple, using something available to everyone: our imagination. Events that we imagine can cause the same physiological changes as "real" events and can have a similarly powerful effect upon our feelings and attitudes. For example, Dr. Antonio Madrid reports thirty cases of children whom he treated for asthma and whose bonding with their mothers had been disrupted at birth. Although Dr. Madrid used several methods of treatment, the major shift occurred when he encouraged the mothers to imagine the kind of loving birth they wished they and their child had shared. The result was that the children's asthma diminished or ceased entirely. This illustrates the power of the imagination to heal not only asthma but also underlying hurts such as disrupted bonding. We and those we care for can be healed when we bring love into our hurtful memories, no matter how deep or how early the trauma.

❧ *Healing Process for Oneself*

This chapter and each one that follows include prayers for healing, called Healing Processes. We use the terms *prayer* and *healing process* interchangeably because we believe that prayer is a process of opening oneself to the healing love of God.

1. Close your eyes and breathe deeply, breathing in the healing love of God, as you understand God.

2. Imagine that you are creating a Christmas crib scene. Imagine that you have all the materials you need to create it in any way you wish. How would you design it, what surroundings, animals or other creatures would you include, and who would be there?

   If you are not Christian, imagine creating the most welcoming birthplace you could wish for. How would you design it; what surroundings, animals, or other creatures would you include; and who would be there?

3. Imagine yourself in the scene you have created. Breathe deeply, breathing in love from the people you have placed there, from the animals or other creatures you have included, and from God.

4. You might wish to draw what you have imagined or to fashion it out of clay, etc., and keep it as a setting for other healing processes that we will suggest throughout this book.

CHAPTER 3

Before Conception

Several times recently, a friend (face full of wonder) has told us a version of the following story:

> A couple had a little girl and a newborn son. The girl kept asking to be alone with the baby. Her parents were afraid to allow it because they thought perhaps she was jealous of her new brother and would harm him. Finally they agreed to the child's request, but they listened in through the intercom in the newborn's room. The girl entered the room and at first all was quiet. Then the parents heard their daughter say to the baby, "Tell me about heaven. I'm beginning to forget."

What impresses us is not only how frequently we hear this same story, but also that so many people claim to know who started it! For example, our friends in North Carolina and in Colorado each assured us that it originated with a local family there.

Why does this story touch people so deeply, and why is it so widespread? At our first workshop of William's, in our group of eighteen, the most common hurt was what William called "divine homesickness," the same as that of the girl in the above story. Divine homesickness refers to a longing for our true home in heaven and a sadness at having had to leave the heart of God, who knew us even before we were in the womb (Jer 1:4–5).

For example, I (Dennis) was born into a family with a vengeful, punitive image of God. During William's workshops, I discovered that I did not want to be born because I was trying to return to the unconditionally loving God I had known. The womb seemed dark in comparison. Even my birth position seems to symbolize this: I was a breech birth (born feet first), perhaps because I was reaching back for the light from which I came.

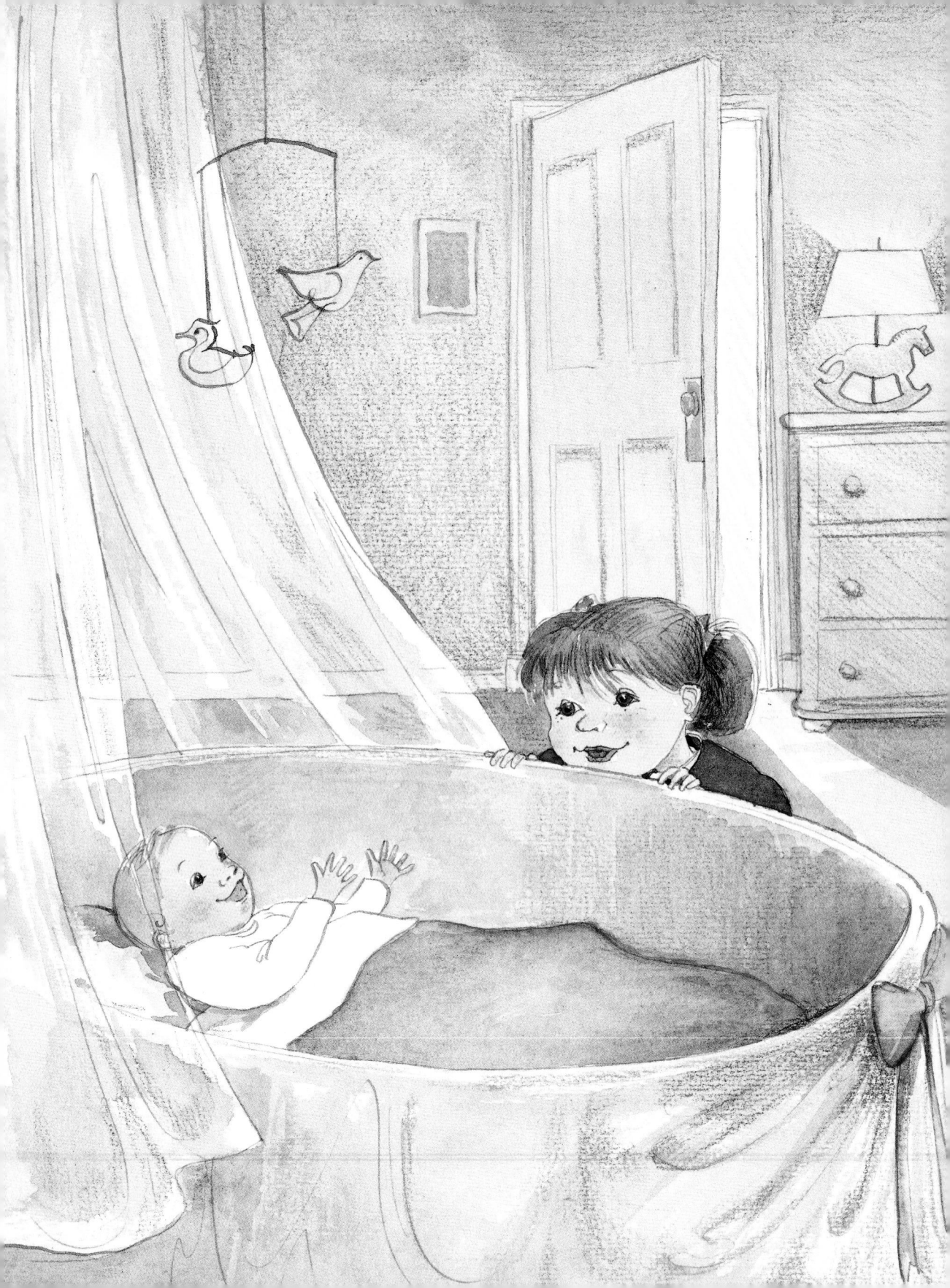

I realized that what had sustained me was communicating with my older brother, Matt, from the moment of conception onward. Often if parents are unable to understand the suffering of a baby in the womb, that baby will seek comfort from young siblings. Matt was two years older than I, and when I was in the womb he had not yet forgotten the heart of God. Psychiatrist Joan Fitzherbert writes that until around the age of two, children are in intimate contact with the mind of God. Their consciousness is only partially here—the rest is with the One from whom they came. Thus, our John is still on his way into this world.

Are Babies Trying to Help Us Remember Our True Home?

Our first words to John were, "We will do all we can to help you remember where you came from." Lately, we've come to suspect that he is saying back to us, "I'm going to do all *I* can to help *you* remember where I came from."

For example, at first we thought John's first spoken word to us was "Hi," but now we think what he has really been saying is "Light." Since early infancy, John's favorite places in the house have been lamps and light switches, which he learned to operate when he was four months old. His favorite toy is a flashlight. Why is John so fascinated by light, often swinging his arms and legs in ecstasy when he sees it? And why, when he is most upset, is it light that comforts him (besides our arms and Sheila's breast)?* A friend who teaches pediatrics told us that fascination with light is very common among babies.

Could it be that light reminds babies of their original home in the heart of God? Light is a universal symbol of God and of heaven. For example, although they vary in other ways, the one detail that the gospel accounts of Jesus' birth have in common is that Jesus brought the light into darkness (Mt 2:2, Lk 2:8–9, Jn 1:5). We traditionally celebrate Christmas on December 25, which ancient people in the Northern

---

*You may wonder what an adopted child is doing at his mother's breast. Actually, it is entirely possible for adoptive mothers to breast-feed, as I (Sheila) did. I first learned about "adoptive nursing" from the popular parenting guide by William and Martha Sears, *The Baby Book: Everything You Need to Know About Your Baby—From Birth to Age Two* (New York: Little, Brown, 1993), pp. 183–184.

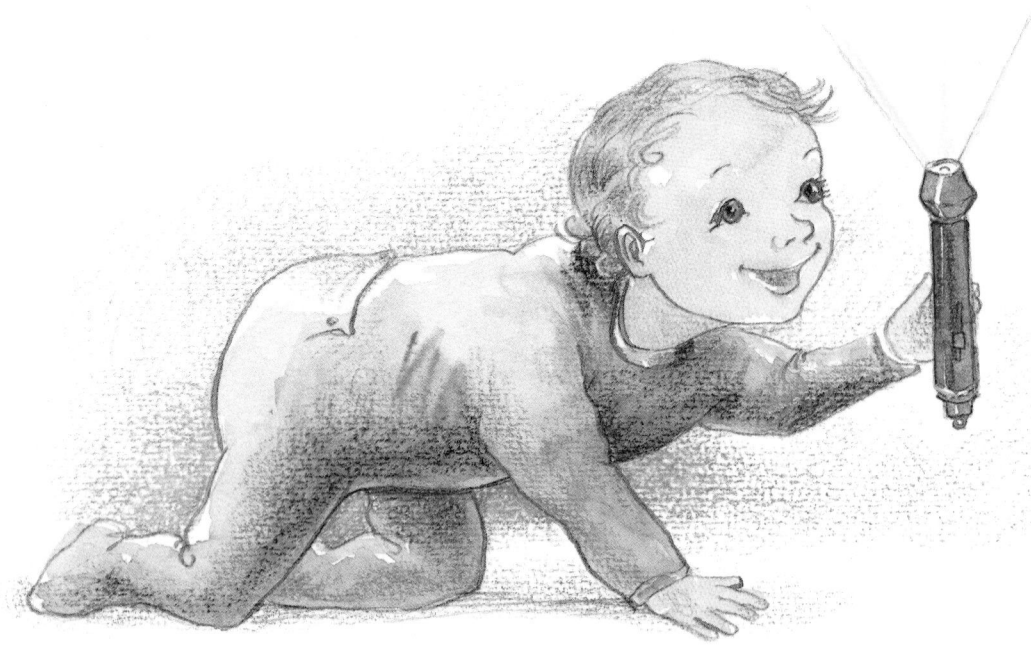

Hemisphere believed was the winter solstice. Thus, while people of other religions prayed for the return of the sun on the darkest night of the year, Christians transformed this custom into praying for the coming of Jesus, the Light of the World. This Christian theme of light is evident today in our use of lights to decorate homes, Christmas trees, Advent wreaths, and so on.

Meeting in the Light

Recently a couple asked us if the best way for them to pray for a child to adopt was to ask God to send them a baby. I (Dennis) responded that the way Sheila and I prayed was to connect ourselves with the baby who was already coming to us. For two years before John's birth, we lit a candle each morning and prayed for the baby who would be ours. I prayed with my breathing: when I exhaled, I would breathe light into our baby, and when I inhaled, I would breathe that baby's light into me. We kept the candle lit all the rest of the day.

When John was three weeks old, Sheila and I brought him with us to our third of William's workshops. During my regression, I expected to feel the same darkness in the womb as during the previous workshops. However, this time the womb was full of light. I realized that it had been there all along, but I had been too traumatized to see it. Now, I knew the light came with me into this world and would never leave me.

At that moment, William brought John to me. I sensed John's spirit join me in the light. He reached out and pulled on my shirt. This was the moment when I first felt bonded to him (unlike Sheila, who had felt bonded to John the moment she met him). It made sense that John would recognize me in the light because it was there that we had already been connected.

Before Conception as a Prenatal Stage

It may seem strange to include the time before conception in a book on healing prenatal and perinatal trauma. We (Dennis, Sheila, and Matt) come from a tradition in which the idea of preexistence (a conscious life before conception) is not theologically orthodox. At the same time, we respect the many years of experience with people in regression that have led William to include the time before conception as a stage of prenatal development.

Perhaps near-death experiences (NDEs) can help us find a way to interpret preconception reports. At least 8 million Americans claim to have had NDEs. Reports of preconception experiences often include similar elements to those reported in NDEs. For example, preconception experiences often include leaving a loving community and a Being of Light and being given a special purpose. NDEs often include being welcomed by a loving community and a Being of Light and being reminded of one's special purpose on Earth.

Some researchers interpret NDEs literally, believing that they are actual experiences of the next life. Others interpret them as projection, meaning that the near-death experience is entirely a symbolic expression of the inner life of the person and tells us nothing about life after death. Still others would say that they are a mixture of the two: authentic glimpses of the next world, but more or less colored by projections of one's own psychological and cultural biases. Similarly, some interpret reports of preconception experiences literally, believing that we do have a conscious life in heaven before we are conceived. Others might interpret such reports in a

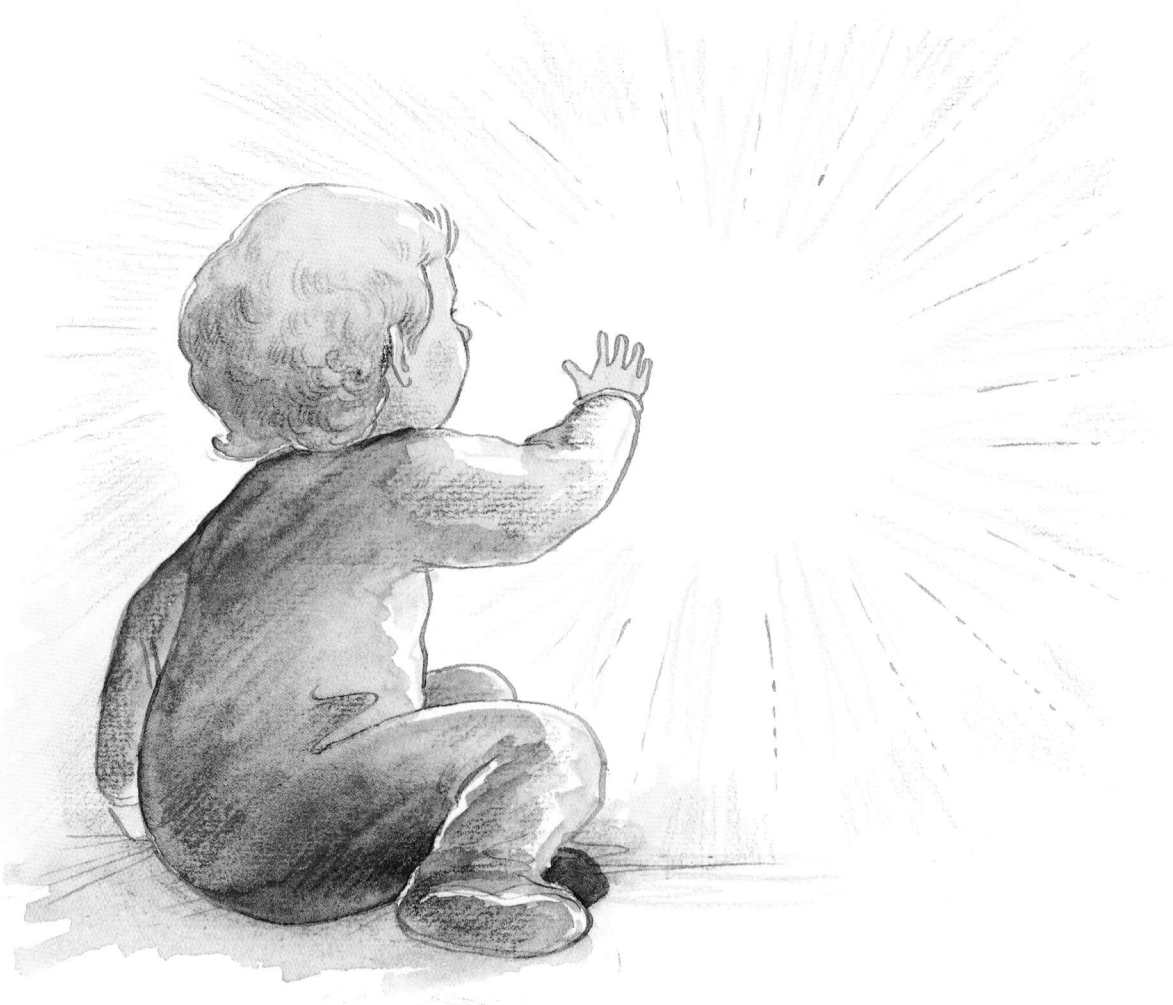

symbolic way, as projection. Within orthodox Christian doctrine, we could say that because we come from the heart of God, we carry within us an awareness of another world that transcends this one, a world that transcends time and our ways of measuring it. Because there is no chronological time in God, God knew us intimately from all eternity, even if we were not yet conscious beings ourselves. What William calls divine homesickness would then be our longing to return to the God who created us at conception. The way that we conceptualize God and our creation would be colored by our own psychological and cultural biases. Regardless of the explanation, preconception experiences invite us to the lifelong task of examining our biases and, most importantly, of saying "Yes" to God and to our life's mission.

Leaving the Heart of God

I (William) have observed that people commonly regress to what they report as the time before conception. The main developmental issue that such people have shared with me is the journey from being spirit to being in a body. They describe this journey in a fairly consistent way that includes a deep understanding of the special purpose of their life and the struggles they will face in living out that purpose. Although the stages of the journey are consistent, the attitude of the journeyer varies considerably.

Some report a wholehearted willingness to be conceived. At the other extreme are those who see themselves as having been "thrown out of heaven" and forced into earthly life. Most people report something in between these two extremes. However literally or symbolically one interprets these reports, they do correlate with how people experience their lives. Thus, for example, although I do not believe that God actually throws anyone out, people who perceive God as having done this to them are likely to live their lives as exiles until their perception of God is healed.

I have observed three types of conception journeys. First are those who recall a willingness to be conceived. They feel little or no disconnection from God and are glad to be here. About 10 percent of people are in this category. Such people tend to live quite happy lives, full of love and caring with relatively little struggle. They seem very connected to their life's destiny and often achieve great things. Simpleness of purpose and of life is characteristic of them.

A second group—60 to 70 percent—report understanding that it was in their best interest to be conceived and that there was a special purpose for their life on earth. At the same time, they say they felt reluctant to leave their life with God. Thus, their process of incorporating into a body, of being in a womb, and of living on earth is marked by feeling a separation from and longing for God. I call this longing divine homesickness.

When divine homesickness remains unconscious and unresolved, life may seem gray and lacking in meaning, and people may be susceptible to various forms of depression. When people consciously identify their divine homesickness and enter a healing process, they often discover that their depression and their longings for money, power, romantic love, and so on are really a longing to reconnect with God. As they realize that God's presence came with them at birth and remains with them, they arrive at a desire to be in this earthly life. They report feeling divine presence in every cell of their bodies, in every action of their minds and every movement of their heart.

The third type of preconception journey is what I call the journey of exile, in which people feel exiled from or cast out of heaven. This occurs about 20 to 30 percent of the time. Until such people find healing, they perceive their transition to earthly life as having been made with intense resistance and against their will. Their lives may include attachment and bonding disorders and any of the symptoms in the second category but to a greater degree.

In its most extreme form, some people who perceive themselves as cast out of heaven don't feel as if they belong with God, nor do they feel that they belong on earth, unless it is with other misfits. They may feel anger and rage at God, which may then be turned against the self. Thus, these "castouts" feel that they must be innately bad or wrong to have been treated as such. Their consciousness may polarize into good and evil, resulting in a deep sense of shame and guilt. At one extreme, they may identify with evil and the devil. Such identification might be acted out through involvement with satanism and ritual abuse. Or, they may go to the opposite extreme and act out by righteously and rigidly campaigning against whomever or whatever they label as evil.

The Significance of Pre-Conception

In terms of life impact, the first wound we experience is always the most important because it exerts the most influence. All other life events are interpreted in terms of the first wounding. In the stage of preconception, the primary wound is separation from God. So, for example, leaving our birth mother and being born may be experienced in a way that parallels how we experienced leaving the heart of God and being conceived into a body. We may experience any other loss in life in a similar way. A job loss, a divorce, or the death of a loved one may feel like the cataclysmic loss of being separated from God, if that was our first wound. Also, if we perceive coming into this world as a disaster, we are likely to view our death in the same way.

I Am Meant To Be

However one interprets the reports of preconception experiences that are described above by William, the basis for a healthy life is to be at peace with God as the one who created us and with our own earthly existence. For example, our friend Joseph had sought for years to heal the wounds of his emotionally deprived childhood. He lived with an underlying uncertainty about the "rightness" of his existence. He also lived with a pervasive fear of death. Although intellectually Joseph was convinced that God does not punish or send people to hell, in his heart he still feared that when he died God would condemn him. During a prayer process, he had the following experience:

> I kept asking over and over, "How did I get here?" I was not asking this in the sense of biology or reproduction but rather existence. I suddenly experienced a shift in which God seemed to give me the answer. I found myself saying, "I am meant to be. I am meant to be *here*." No matter what the deficiencies of my parents, no matter what the external circumstances, I knew that I was meant to be. God intends and confirms my existence.
>
> This was the most significant spiritual experience of my life. Although I had already experienced much healing of the pain of my childhood, I was still unconsciously waiting for this confirmation of my existence. After this experience, I felt brand new. I felt a desire to affirm my own existence by returning to the use of my middle name, Joseph. I felt like an important, unique part of God's plan and creation.

A surprising result of this experience for Joseph was that he no longer feared death. He told us, "I was meant by God to be, so surely God will see me safely through death." As Joseph discovered, the foundation for healing in our lives (and in our deaths) is a grateful awareness that "I am meant to be."

Once we know this, we can choose life, and our particular life. We experience ourselves as fundamentally good, and we perceive everything else that way, too. We know that all creation came from God and will return to God. Ultimately we arrive at St. Ignatius's goal of "finding the presence of God in all things."

 ## *Healing Process for Oneself*

We begin many of the healing prayers in this book by inviting you to light a candle. If you are a Christian, the candle might be a reminder that, as John 1:9 tells us, Jesus is the light of the world and, as Matthew 5:14 tells us, you are, too. If you are not a Christian, the candle might be a reminder of the light of God (however you understand God) within you.

1. Light a favorite candle.

2. Close your eyes and breathe deeply. Imagine yourself in the safe and welcoming birthplace you created for yourself at the end of Chapter 2.

3. Now imagine yourself going all the way back to the beginning of your existence in the heart of God. Imagine God asking if you would be willing to come into this world.

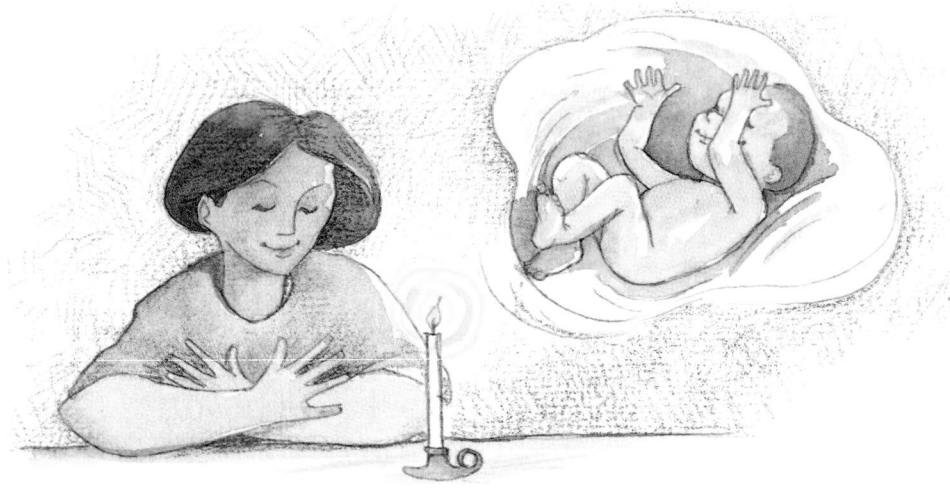

4. Ask yourself, "Do I want to come?" and listen within your whole being for the answer.

5. If your answer is "Yes," imagine yourself coming into this world, enfolded in the loving light of God.

   Then ask yourself, "What would help me enter even more fully into life?" Imagine yourself receiving what you need as you breathe in God's creative and loving light.

6. If your answer is "No," ask yourself, "What would help me become willing to come here?" Perhaps you will think of a special person whose love would help you, a safe place in nature, an activity that gives your life meaning, and so on. Whatever your answer, imagine yourself receiving what you need as you breathe in God's creative and loving light.

℘ *Healing Actions for Oneself*

You might wish to follow up this prayer in these ways:

1. Swing on a swing. (Remember Sheila's rocking chair?) As you go backward, imagine that you are reaching back for your home in the heart of God. As you go forward, bring that home with you into this world.

2. Light a candle at dinner. Let the candle remind you of how the light of God has come with you, and let the dinner be a celebration.

3. Sit in a chair or on the floor. Ask someone you love and trust to stand behind you. Reach your arms straight out in back of your head as far as you can, imagining that you are reaching back for the love of God from which you came. After a short time, ask the person in back of you to take your hands and hold them securely for a while.

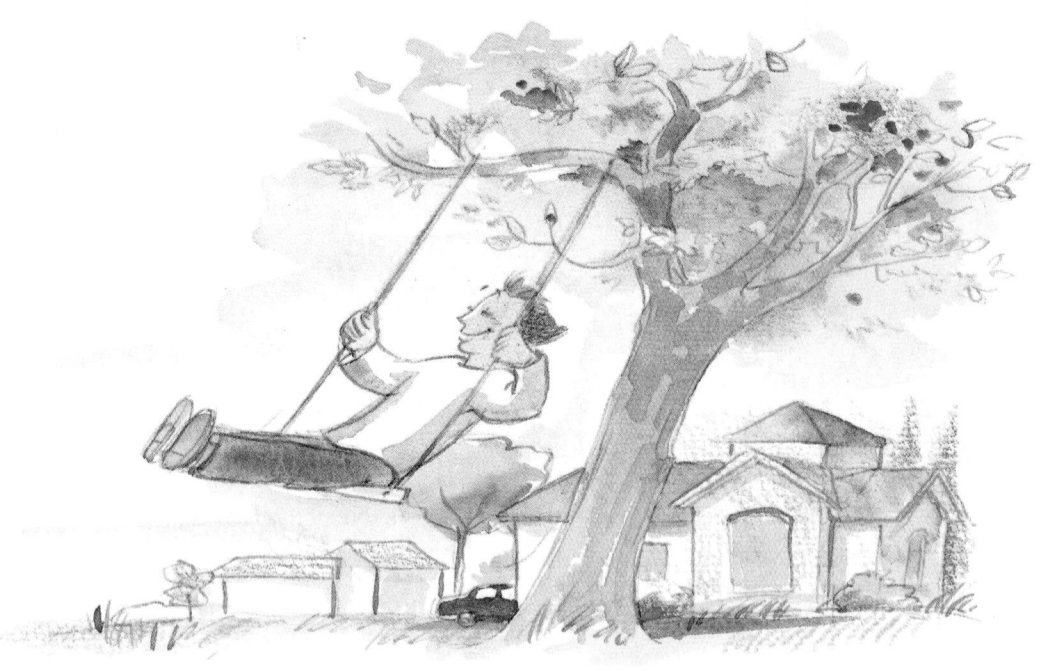

⟡ *Healing Process for Unborn Children*

As mentioned in Chapter 1, a parent's trauma affects babies to the extent that it is unresolved and unconscious. A parent who is not at peace with his or her own existence will pass this dis-ease on to a child. An example of this is a father whose adolescent daughter had always been rebellious and disobedient. She referred to herself as a "bad girl who should be thrown out." Nothing in her parents' relationship to her nor anything in her life seemed to justify the way she felt. The father sought help from a therapist who suggested that he regress back to any scene in his life that would help him understand his daughter.

To his surprise, he perceived himself as back in the period before conception. He perceived himself as having been thrown out of heaven, feeling that he was bad and deserving to be cast out. He realized that his daughter had absorbed his perception of himself as having been exiled and was acting it out. He relived the experience of divine exile five or six times, each time praying for healing. As he did so, not only did he feel better about himself, but this healing was passed on to his daughter, who gradually stopped behaving like a "bad girl."

If you are planning to conceive or adopt a child, you may wish to do the following prayer. You can also pray this prayer for a baby already born or even for grown children.

1. Go back to the Healing Process for Oneself, above. Recall your answer to the question, "Do I want to come?"

2. Focus your attention on the child in the heart of God who will be yours. Wait until you feel your heart move, and then express your honest love and desire for this child. Even if your child has not yet been conceived, your love will reach your child who is in God, in whom there is no time.

3. Now tell your child about your answer to the question, "Do I want to come?"

4. Remind your child that your answer is *yours*, and that he or she need not have the same experience or give the same answer. If you feel unhealed at this stage, assure your child that you will take responsibility to seek healing for yourself.

5. Thank your child for listening and for coming to you. Invite your child to have a safe journey into your family.

◉ *Preconception Game*

Children are always attempting to resolve their pre- and perinatal trauma, most often through play. For example, many children like to crawl through tunnels or go down slides as a way of recapitulating their passage through the birth tunnel. Following is a game for parents and other caring adults to use who want to help children resolve trauma from the preconception stage. This game is especially helpful for three- to six-year-olds, but it can be used with younger or older children as well.

1. Tell your child a story about where children come from, not in the biological sense but in the spiritual sense and in a way that fits your value system and religious beliefs. For example, in a Christian family the story might begin with something like, "Once upon a time, long, long ago, God dreamed of you as our

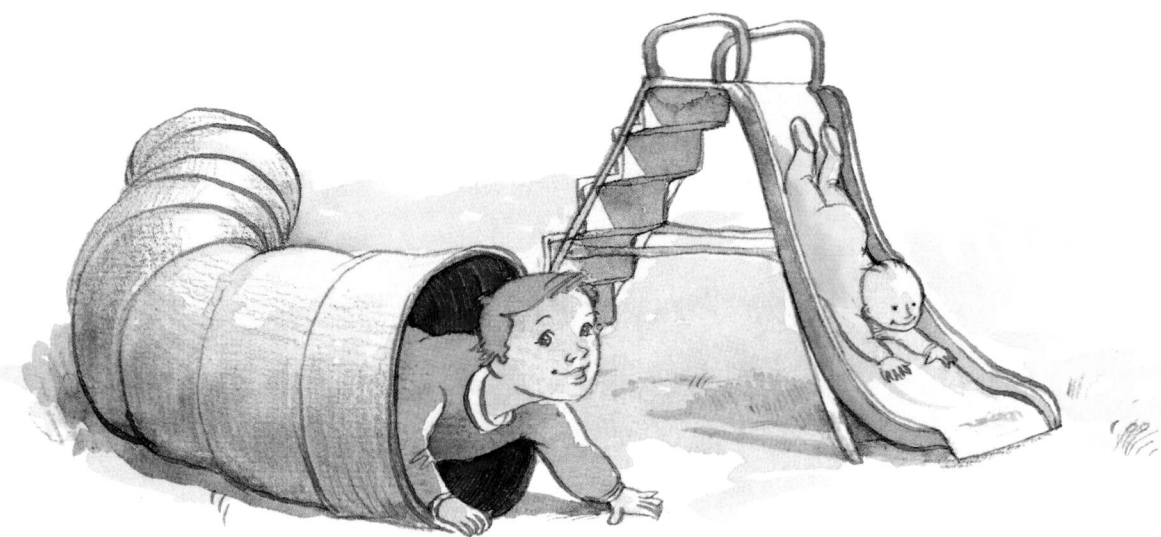

child. . . ." The story should describe where children come from as a magical place, inhabited by wondrous figures such as angels.

2. Place your child in a blanket, and rock the child back and forth for fifteen minutes, carrying the child through darkened hallways into the living room, which symbolizes earth.

3. As you carry the child, tell him or her that they are going to earth. Ask the child to say goodbye to the place from which he or she came. Ask how the child feels about coming closer to earth, about meeting family members, and so on.

Make the game fun and follow the leads of the child. For example, some children like to play spinning games, wear special clothes or costumes, draw pictures, decorate the living room, and so on before or during the game. Allow the expression of all kinds of feelings, and mirror the feelings back to the child. Also allow rapid body movements, kicking, dancing, singing, crying, laughing, and so on.

Note: As in this chapter, each of the following chapters will conclude with a healing process for children and a game that adults can play with children. Both will be healing to the extent that adults are empathically present to children. One simple way to enhance empathic presence is for an adult to match his or her breathing to that of a child. The healing processes and games can be repeated many times with the same child as a way of allowing the healing to deepen. Adults can also play these games with one another in situations designed for healing.

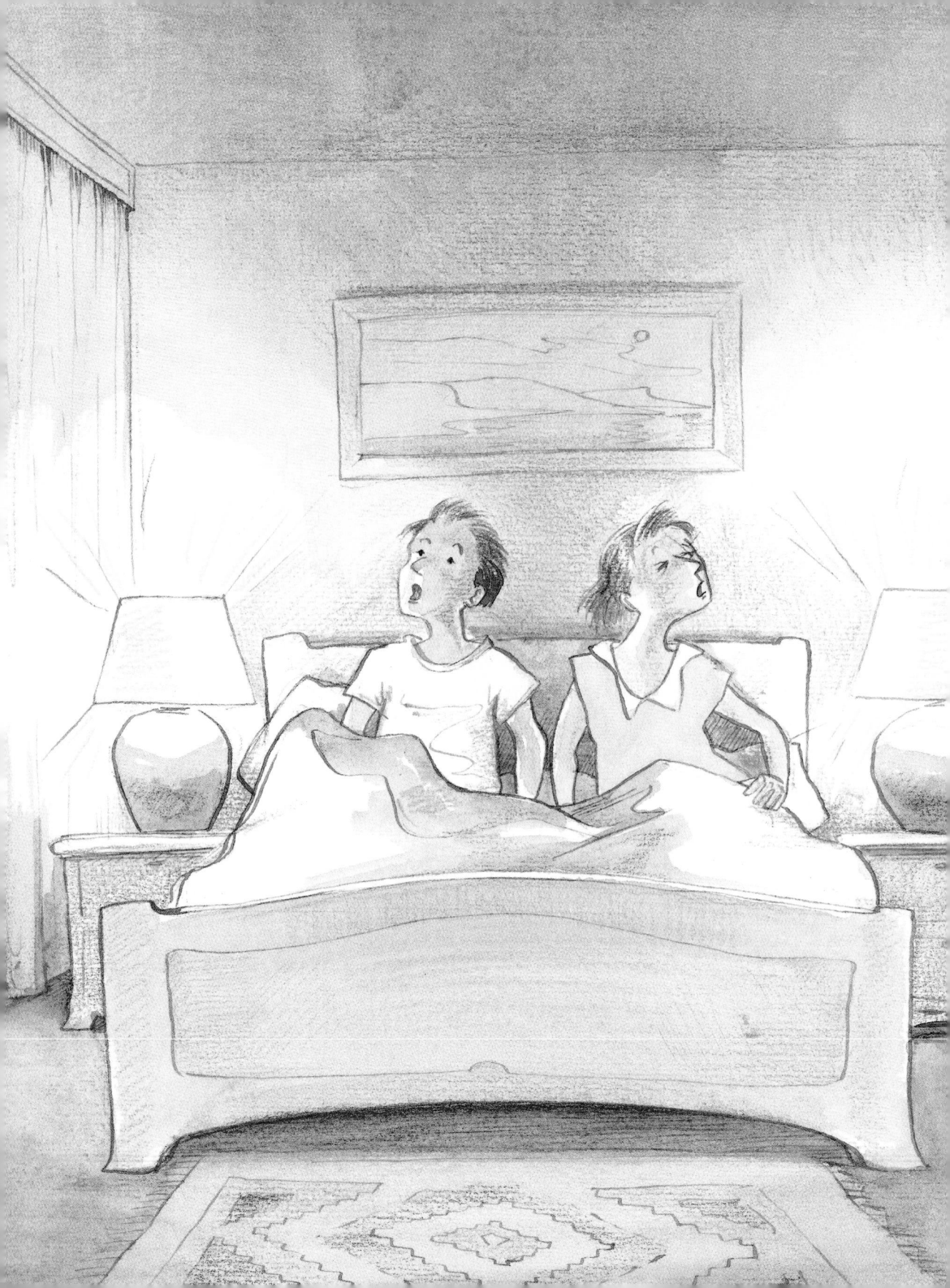

CHAPTER 4

Conception

At its best, conception is a joyful union of egg and sperm in a biochemical explosion of light. All three participants (mother, father, and child) are saying a wholehearted "Yes!" Consider the following story, incredible as it may seem.

Karen and her daughter and son-in-law, Emily and Steve, were on vacation at a resort. At 3:00 A.M., Emily and Steve, faces ashen, knocked on Karen's door. They asked Karen if the lights had gone on in her room. Karen said "No. What's wrong?" Emily and Steve explained they were awakened by the feeling of someone running across the bed. At first, each thought the other was getting up. At the same moment, all the lights went on in the room. The lights were on separate switches, which meant that someone would have had to go from one switch to another to turn them all on at once. As Karen, Emily, and Steve talked about this, Emily sensed that she had conceived a child. Sure enough, Sarah was born nine months later.

Two years after Sarah's birth, the whole family (including Sarah) was together in Karen's kitchen. They recalled the resort vacation. Sarah said, "I remember that place." Her mother said, "How can you remember it? You weren't born yet." Sarah answered, "I was there. Don't you remember? I ran across your bed." No one had ever mentioned to Sarah what had awakened Emily and Steve that evening; yet Sarah apparently remembered her eagerness to be their child. Two years later, Sarah again referred to the evening of her conception. She said, "I was light and I wanted to put more light into the room."

Memories of Conception and Nonlocal Communication

How is this possible? How could Sarah remember her conception? How could she be conceived in Emily's body and seem to run across the bed at the same time? For that matter, how could we (Dennis and Sheila) connect with our son, John, for two years before he came to us at the age of eleven days?

Perhaps recent scientific studies can help us. Highly reputable institutions, such as Stanford and Princeton Universities, are finding that all of us have the capacity for nonlocal communication, meaning communication that transcends space (our physical bodies) and time (the present moment). Dr. Larry Dossey writes,

> For about a decade, studies done at Princeton University's Engineering Anomalies Research Laboratory have indicated that subjects can influence the outcome of random physical events and can mentally convey complex information to other subjects from whom they are widely separated, even by global distances. These studies show not only that a sender can mentally transmit detailed information to a receiver on the other side of the earth, but also that the receiver usually "gets" the information up to three days before it is sent.

At this point, you may be thinking, "Now this is becoming *really* weird!" How can information possibly be received up to three days before it is sent? A clue comes from studies showing that those who are most effective at nonlocal communication are those who are most loving and compassionate. This should not surprise us because when we love we are united with the mind of God, who is love, and God transcends space and time. As we mentioned earlier, it seems that young children are in constant close contact with the mind of God and therefore perhaps especially capable of nonlocal communication.

Another thing that may help us to understand Sarah's experience and some of the other stories that follow is the concept of energy fields that enfold our physical body. This has long been understood in Eastern medicine and is gradually influencing Western medicine, where many reputable health-care professionals are beginning to incorporate therapies based on energy fields into their practices. An example is massage combined with therapeutic touch, which is now accepted to the extent that some insurance companies will pay for it.

The idea behind such therapies is that energy fields (visible through Kirilian photography) surround our physical body and contain all its information. The physical body flows from these energy fields (rather than vice versa). Thus, at the moment of conception, we have an energetic body, even though physically we have only one cell. This energy body is palpable (as Sarah's was to her parents on the night of her conception).

The energy body may help us understand how Sarah could remember events that occurred at the stage of conception. Not long ago, medical science taught that a child could not remember before the age of two because his or her central nervous system was too immature. Today, however, there are several theories to explain how a fetus can remember, even as far back as conception. The research of famed neuroscientist Candace Pert indicates that cells throughout the body are capable of memory through the mechanism of neuropeptides (information molecules manufactured by nerve cells) and their receptors. There are so many receptors in the brain stem that it can be considered part of the limbic system, which plays a key role in memory. Because the brainstem is visible at four weeks from conception, this can provide one explanation for very early memory.

Pert and others go further, however, and suggest that there is an immaterial basis for memory. For example, Rupert Sheldrake's theory is that memory is not really in the brain; rather, memory is in a field that surrounds us, and our brains are like TV receivers that tune in to that field. The research on nonlocal communication described earlier and on nonordinary states of consciousness such as near-death experiences (in which people leave their brain and body and remember information they acquired while they were gone) seem to support the idea that memory is non-physical and spiritual in nature and thus is not confined to the brain. This would explain how memory can go all the way back to conception, when the child has a fully conscious spirit but as yet has no brain.

My (William's) experience confirms that memories of unresolved trauma are stored in the energy field that surrounds the physical body. These memories can be located and activated by trained persons, and I have done this for thirty years. We (Dennis and Sheila) have been learning to do this. We are astonished at its effectiveness in treating preverbal children, as well as adults who cannot consciously remember their early trauma. Effective diagnosis and treatment through energy fields of people who have unresolved trauma relies on a loving relationship between therapist and patient. Our belief is that in healing prayer, which is based upon love, traumas can be touched and healed even when we don't know how to locate them.

Healing Birth Trauma
Develops Compassion and Boundaries

Back to Sarah. Although Sarah's conception and prenatal life were surrounded by love, her birth was difficult because her left shoulder was caught in the birth canal. As an infant, she received treatment for this. Treatment includes empathically verbalizing for a baby what he or she may have felt during a traumatic experience. Although parents and other caregivers may not be trained in all the techniques of treating children with prenatal and perinatal trauma, any loving person can empathically verbalize for a child what that child may have felt.

Because treatment is based upon empathic presence, one of the great benefits of treatment in early life is that it models and encourages the natural capacity for empathy in children. The first eighteen months are especially critical for the development of empathy, and it is especially beneficial for a child to receive intense empathic presence during this time, as Sarah did.

For example, when Sarah was ten months old, she and her grandmother, Karen, were eating in a restaurant. A mother came in with a baby boy who was having a tantrum. Sarah crawled over, sat down in front of the boy, and imitated his behavior. She made eye contact with him and maintained it. The boy began to calm down. Sarah smiled at him and he smiled back. His mother realized what had happened and, referring to Sarah, said, "That's empathy!" Thus, while unresolved prenatal and perinatal trauma can harm a child's emotional development, if that trauma is resolved, the child can become extraordinarily compassionate and empathic.

Besides empathy, another result of healing prenatal and perinatal trauma is the ability to maintain healthy boundaries. For example, when Sarah was ten months old, her father (whom she loves and trusts and who encourages Sarah to have healthy boundaries) reached out to touch her. Sarah, who did not want to be touched at that moment, removed his hand from her body and said, "No touch me now!" If Sarah could establish such a clear boundary at ten months, she will likely be able to protect herself from violation and intrusion later in life. Intrusion includes all forms of unwanted touch, including sexual abuse.

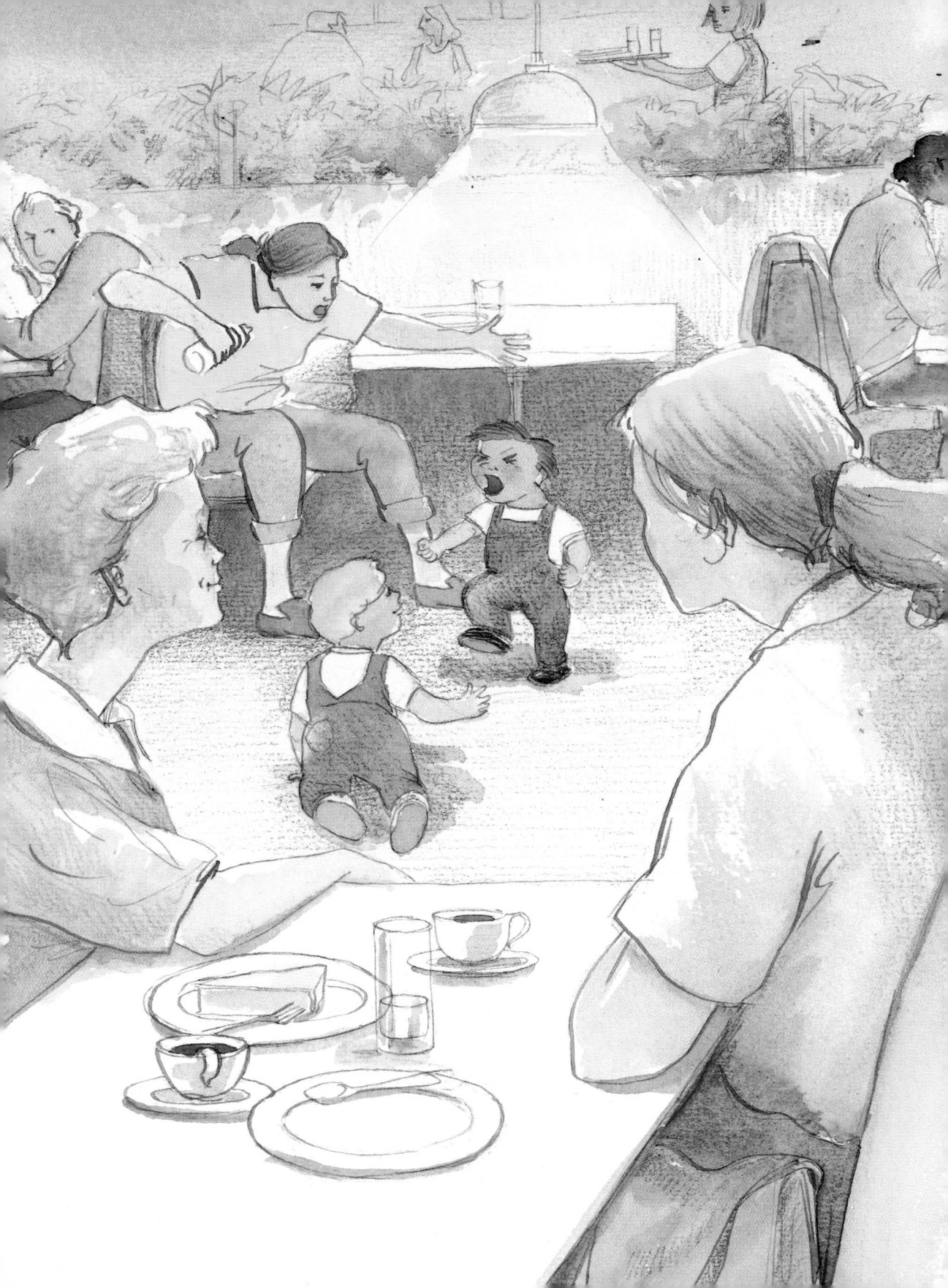

Like Sarah, people who resolve prenatal and perinatal trauma can say "Yes" and "No" in situations where they formerly experienced themselves as helpless victims of forces beyond their control. For example, in contrast to Sarah, I (Sheila) have always been easily intimidated by people whom I experience as intrusive or overwhelming, and I was not able to protect myself from sexual abuse as a child. During one birth regression, I recalled times when I felt invaded to such an extent that I experienced it as life threatening.

As I breathed into this experience, I noticed a tight feeling in my throat as if I were being suffocated. My hands were facing each other several inches apart, and they began to move back and forth toward each other. I felt something between them that was palpably thick, like gelatin. Then I collapsed and began to gasp. I felt desolate and helpless.

The therapist working with me, Laura, told me that I had just experienced conception. She said that when a woman is afraid of intercourse and of conceiving (as my mother was), the egg emits a thick substance to keep the sperm away . . . like gelatin. Laura encouraged me to push away what was coming at me and say "No!" At first, my "No" was a bare whisper, but as Laura lovingly encouraged me to continue, my "No" grew to a loud and emphatic "NO!" that came from the center of my body. Since then I have felt a clear space within from which I am better able to set boundaries and protect myself from intrusion without fear.

My mother was extremely frightened of sexuality. This early experience of my mother's fear apparently imprinted upon me and left me feeling helpless to say "No." I was then vulnerable to sexual abuse as an older child. I now had two layers of wounding related to intrusion. This layering of wounding is typical in that unhealed prenatal and perinatal trauma creates the template mentioned earlier on which subsequent and related traumatic experiences build up in layers.

Symptoms of Conception Trauma

Sarah's and Sheila's stories exemplify how profoundly the moment of conception can affect us and set the tone for the rest of life. But can we actually remember this moment? In Chapter 1, I (William) described the challenge it was for me to trust my memories of my birth. As I began my career of accompanying others who were having spontaneous memories of their births, I faced an even greater challenge.

People began to regress spontaneously to their prenatal life and even to their conception. They consistently reported to me their memories of being sperm and egg and of experiencing the union of the two.

To research this further, I spent about 200 hours in elementary school classrooms, asking second- and third-graders to draw pictures of what it was like to be inside their mothers when their bodies were made. The children drew pictures that were consistent with embryological facts, including structures that looked like ovaries and tubes and the egg and sperm coming together. This led me to believe that memories of conception are innate. Such memories are typically repressed by the rational adult mind but can be recovered through regression.

My friend and colleague, Dr. Graham Farrant, experienced this. Until his death, Graham was a pioneer in the fields of cellular research and of healing prenatal and perinatal trauma. During a regression experience of his own in 1979, which was recorded on videotape, two elements contradicted medical knowledge of conception at that time. First, Graham experienced the egg opening two "arms" to embrace a chosen sperm. Second, he experienced the fertilized egg hesitating in the fallopian tube, as if uncertain whether or not to go on.

Four years later, in 1983, the Karolinska Institute released the film "Miracle of Life," which showed the actual process of conception. Graham played this film side by side with the videotape of his 1979 regression. His own spontaneous movements during regression mirrored exactly what actually takes place during conception and what is now accepted medically. For example, contrary to the common perception that the sperm always aggressively penetrates the egg, we now know that the egg can actively participate in choosing and welcoming a particular sperm into itself. Similarly, we now know that the fertilized egg can hesitate on its journey down the fallopian tube.

The degree of consciousness that a child has at conception is illustrated by two children from different families. Although the most obvious symptoms were interpersonal problems, I discovered that in each case the child was irrationally obsessed with temperature. One child was intensely interested in cold. All he could talk about was going to live in Alaska, as if that was the only safe and meaningful place on Earth. One whole wall of his room was covered with pictures of ice-capped mountains. The other child had an aversion to cold. She felt cold all the time and couldn't get warm. All she could talk about was going to live in a tropical environment.

As it turned out, both of these children came from frozen embryos. One was directly recapitulating his experience by continually seeking cold, and the other was avoidantly recapitulating her experience by continually seeking warmth. In both cases, the experience of being frozen had affected the child's trust of the parents, and it was this distrust that was being acted out in family conflicts. After a couple of treatment sessions during which the child expressed what it was like to be frozen, in each case the child became relaxed about temperature. Simultaneously, the family conflicts diminished.

From such experiences and from reports of memories of conception that thousands of people in addition to Graham have shared with me, I've formed a picture of what happens. The child who is being conceived experiences his or her own unique spirit as given by God. The child's spirit participates in the consciousness of the sperm and the egg and in the relationship between the parents. The child thus has a direct experience of the sperm and the egg that led to the formation of his or her body.

The Sperm Journey

The experiences of the sperm and its journey toward the egg that have been reported to me typically include a life-and-death struggle. This is consistent with the work of an embryologist who measured the length of a sperm and the distance from the scrotum to the fallopian tube (where most babies are conceived). Given the size of a sperm, its journey is comparable to an adult having to swim almost 400 miles through many life-threatening situations in which nearly all its millions of companions will die.

The sperm journey includes a sense of fraternity and unity of purpose with the other sperm. Recent embryological research has confirmed this and has discovered that sperm are like bees and ants. Particular groups of sperm have special functions

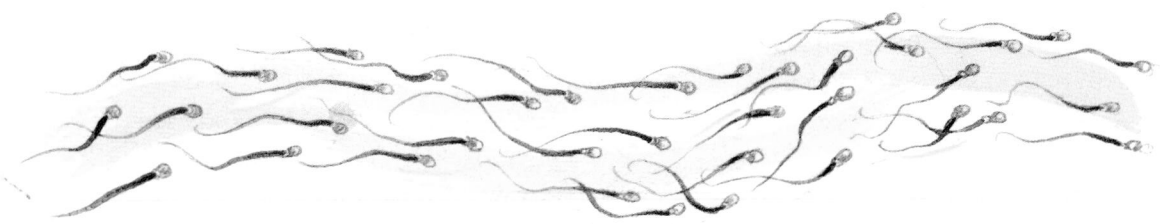

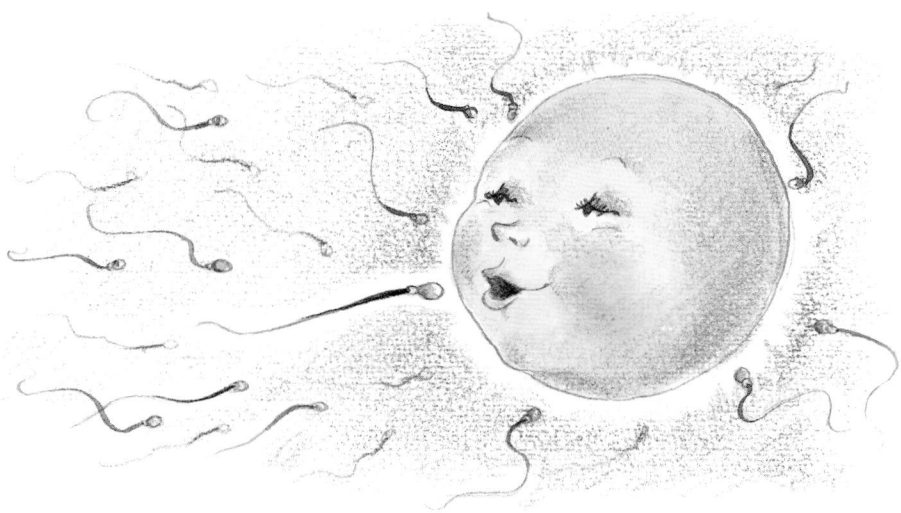

for the survival of the whole species. Some provide latticework so they can cross crevices and chasms; others provide protective barriers against the immune system of the mother; and so on. Sperm exhibit an incredible degree of intelligence in their interworking as they pursue their one purpose.

Despite their efforts to cooperate, the sperm recognize that most will die. They are fighting together against very high biological odds, even in a loving and receptive human body. At the point when the egg is in sight, all the remaining sperm turn themselves toward the final goal. The main theme at this stage is competitiveness. There's first place, maybe second place, and occasionally third place. I suspect that many people recapitulate this through such things as causes and crusades, theatrical productions involving tragedy and heroism, and sports. For example, sports events, with teams involved in win/loss situations as they pursue a round ball, can provide a healthy way of reenacting the sperm journey and of grieving its losses.

The final stage of the sperm journey is the attainment and penetration of the egg. If the relationship between the parents is not good and/or the mother's body is not welcoming, the sperm may perceive the egg as engulfing (it's thousands of times bigger than any one sperm), all-powerful, and annihilating. If the parents' relationship is loving and the mother is welcoming, the egg is likely to be perceived as powerful but good. The sperm then go to the egg willingly and even ecstatically, happy to complete their biological mission.

When a sperm enters an egg, the head enters first. Then the tail loses its power and drops off. The head explodes and the sperm is literally consumed by the egg. Thus, instant success is followed by loss of one's identity and one's life and by being consumed for another's purpose. Although men and women carry within them memories of both the sperm and the egg journeys, men tend to identify more with the journey of the sperm and women tend to identify more with that of the egg. I believe that the experience of being consumed by the egg is a major biological basis of commitment–anxiety in men. Many men are afraid to commit themselves to women for fear of losing their identity. Many women experience men as unable to commit themselves, as "wanting only sex but not my heart."

If, however, conception was wholesome and loving or if any hurts from the sperm journey have been healed, we bring with us gifts from the sperm. These gifts include the ability to persist in reaching a goal, enjoying the camaraderie of others, taking initiative, acceptance of death, and the capacity for union.

The Egg Journey

Unlike sperm, which have a short life-span, eggs have lived together for many years, beginning when the mother was a fetus in the body of the grandmother. Their first experience during conception is leaving their sorority or sisterhood. This leaving involves both grief and loss.

The egg then drops out of the ovary into seemingly vast space. This imprints instinctual fear of loss of control and of falling. Later fears of taking risks and initiative and of being on one's own begin here. Suctional forces then draw the egg up into the fallopian tube. The experience of being pulled up in this way is like being rescued. The fallopian tube is a safer space in which a milky substance feeds and propels the egg.

As Graham Farrant experienced, the egg participates in choosing a particular sperm. Nevertheless, if the relationship between the parents is not good and if the mother's body is not safe, the egg may perceive sperm as a gang intent on rape. However, if the parental relationship is good and the mother's body is safe, the egg may perceive the sperm as powerful and may experience fear, but it nevertheless willingly welcomes the sperm.

If conception was wholesome and loving or if hurts from the egg journey have

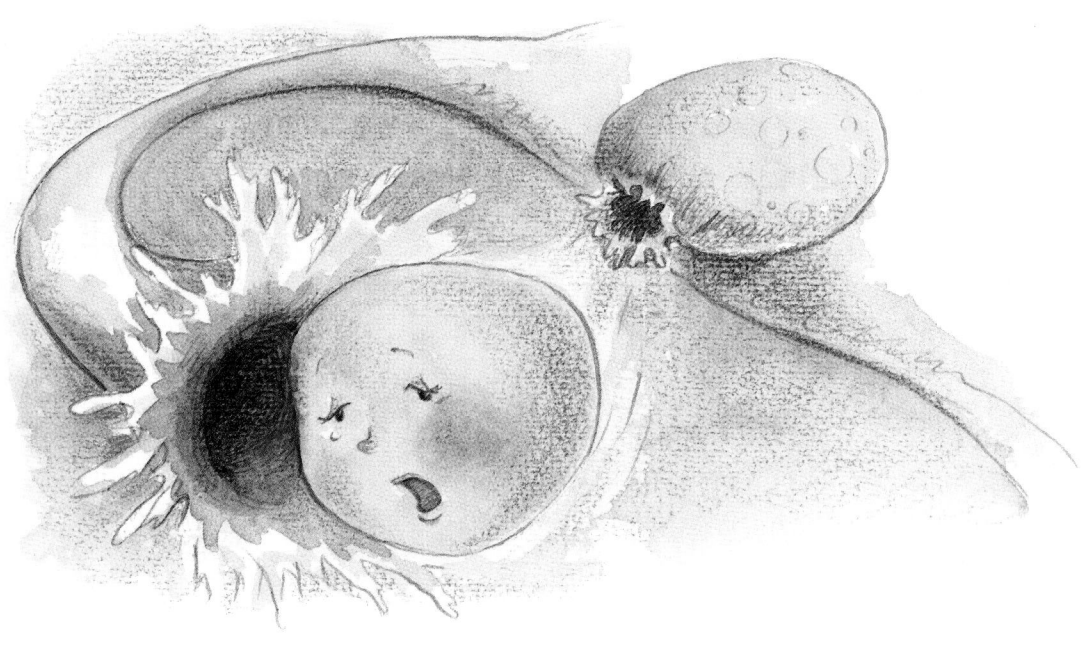

been healed, we bring with us special gifts from the egg. These gifts include the ability to stay inside oneself and to be introspective, to value procreation, to enjoy women as friends, to trust help from above and to accept rescuing and help, to cooperate and to take risks with conscious vulnerability.

The Parents' Relationship

The child is aware not only of the experiences of the sperm and egg but also of the relationship between the parents. Thus, if there is violence between the parents, the child experiences his or her conception as fundamentally aggressive and violent. If the parents are involved in drug abuse, the child's experience of conception includes diffusiveness, loss of orientation, and loss of vitality. (Moreover, according to research by T. J. Cicero and others, the use of cigarettes, alcohol, or other drugs prior to conception by either parent can harm the sperm or the egg.) If the parents' sexual relationship includes sexual shame, the child's memory of conception is infused with shame and guilt. If a baby is conceived accidentally or is unwanted, the baby has intimate contact with that knowledge. Conversely, if a child is conceived by parents who love and respect one another and who want that child, the foundation has been laid in the child for self-respect and the ability to give and receive love.

Relationships Between Men and Women

Men and women who go through the resolution of conception trauma understand each other better. In our culture, we often assume that antagonism between the sexes is inevitable. The popular saying, "women are from Venus and men are from Mars," presumes that men and women are virtually two different species who have vastly different experience and desires. However, the fact that both genders carry memories of the sperm and the egg journeys gives a new dimension to Jung's insight that we all have both masculine and feminine aspects of identity within ourselves. It also means that men and women *are* capable of understanding one another. As people resolve their conception trauma, they often find a new capacity to integrate masculine and feminine within and to understand the opposite sex and to relate to them as friends.

Conception and Spirituality

In Western culture, it is commonly believed that babies in the early stages of prenatal development are minimally conscious or not conscious at all. As mentioned in Chapter 1, it is assumed that human beings grow in consciousness as they mature, and in one sense this is correct. However, as we have said, the opposite is also true. A baby at the moment of conception has a spirit created by God. This spirit is fully conscious of life and of God and has not yet experienced many of the hurts that cause human beings to defend themselves and shut down their spiritual awareness. Our challenge at conception was to maintain contact with our own unique spirit and with the unlimited love of God. We struggled to do this even as we merged with matter, in all its limitations.

Christian spirituality recapitulates this in the sacraments. Through the use of created things, such as the water of baptism, the oil of anointing the sick, or the bread and wine of Eucharist, every sacrament ritualizes the union of spirit and matter that we all experienced at conception. Christian spirituality also recapitulates the union of spirit and matter in its assertion that Jesus was conceived of the Holy Spirit (rather than through sexual intercourse). Aside from its doctrinal significance, the biblical story of Jesus' conception (the Annunciation) symbolizes the human desire to maintain contact with the Spirit as we merged with matter at conception.

In addition to the challenge of merging with matter, from conception our fully conscious spirits were marinated in the inner lives of our parents, with all their hurts. Christian spirituality calls this marinade original sin. Because there is no chronological time in God, in prayer we can transmit loving influences now to the conceptus we were then. That is why, as Christians, we say that baptism can take away many of the effects of original sin.

Because our consciousness at conception was so vast, we could take in not only hurts but also love wherever it was offered. Thus, although our (Dennis and Sheila's) son John was exposed to extremely destructive influences during

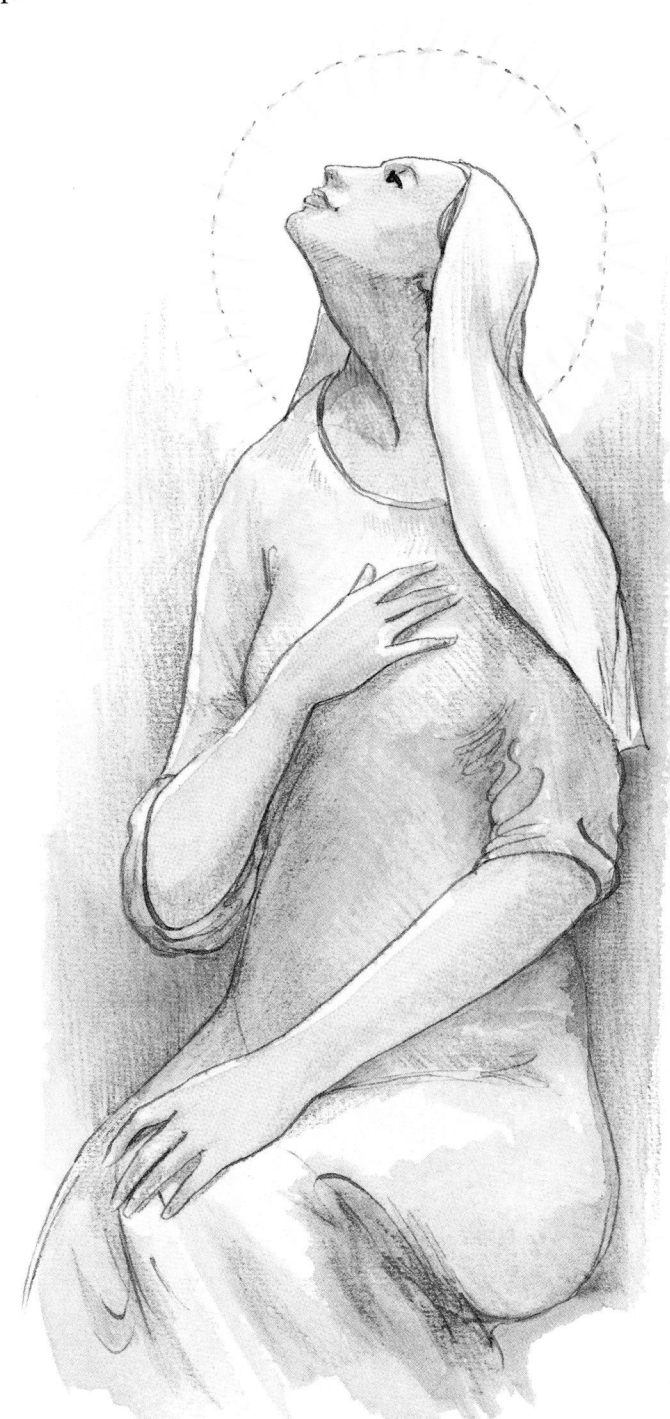

his conception and gestation, he is an entirely healthy and loving child. We believe that this is because so many people were praying with us for him, because his spirit took in those prayers (and still does), and because of his courageous work on his prenatal and perinatal traumas.

❧ *Healing Process for Oneself*

In the Annunciation, the angel Gabriel proclaims to Mary that she will conceive a special child. She says "Yes"—she chooses him. Soon Joseph, too, will choose Jesus. In the following prayer, we invite Mary to hold us in her body at the moment of our

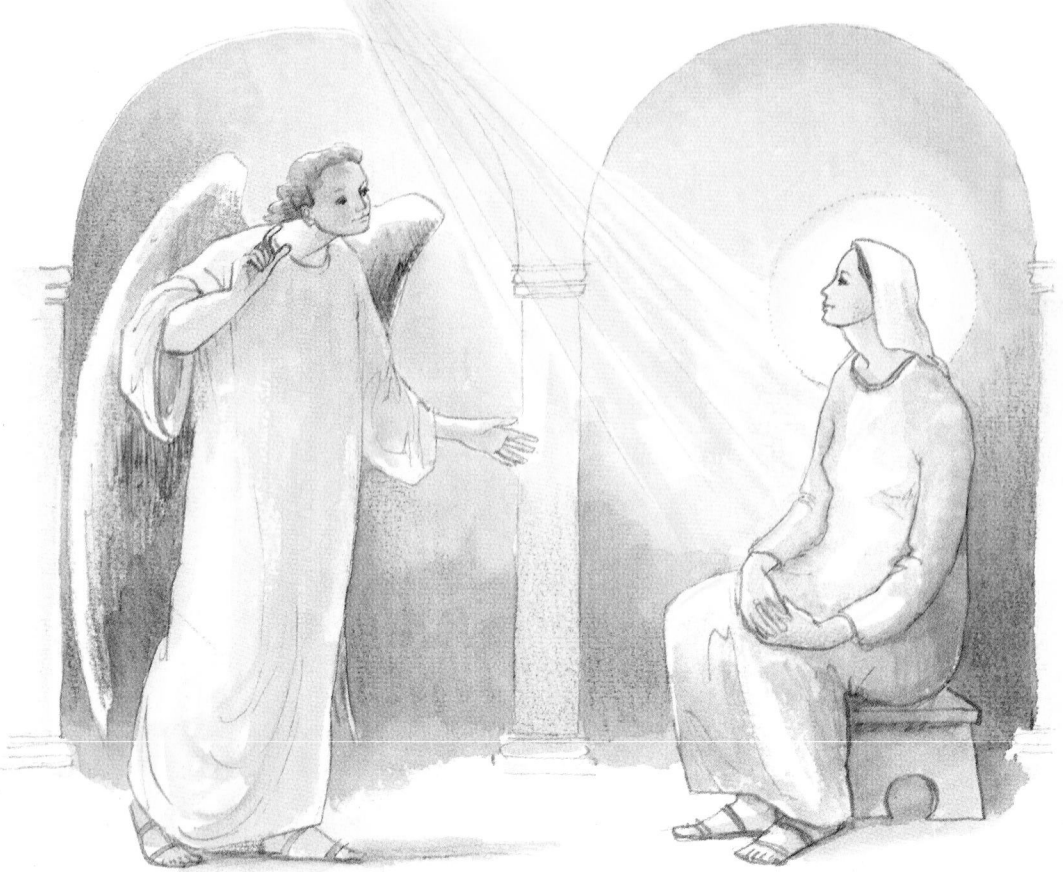

conception. We do this trusting that Mary and Joseph's love is more powerful than whatever negative influences we took in and that their love transcends time and space. If you are not a Christian and/or you are not comfortable praying with Mary, you can do this prayer by imagining yourself in the body of the most loving woman you know. You can also imagine the protective presence of the most loving man you know.

As preparation for this healing prayer process, you may wish to count backward from your birth date to the probable date of your conception. Trust that there is a good reason for whatever date comes to you. Then ask yourself the following questions:

- What significant life events have happened during the month when you were conceived?
- How do you normally feel during this month? Do you feel or act any differently during this month than at other times?
- What two or three words would you use to describe this month?
- Do you prefer or dislike your conception month?

Take a few moments to be with the feeling in your body as you reflect on these questions before doing the following prayer:

1. You may wish to begin by lighting a candle and reading Luke 1:26–38, the Annunciation story.

2. Close your eyes and breathe deeply. Once again, count backward from your birth date to the probable date of your conception.

3. Now, ask yourself what it was like to be conceived in the body of your mother. What was it like for your spirit to merge with matter? To merge with your father's sperm? To merge with your mother's egg? To merge with the relationship between your parents? What did you most need?

4. Let your mother's body become the body of Mary. Imagine Mary resting her hands on the place in her body where you are being conceived. Imagine Joseph standing protectively by her, with his hands over hers. Breathe in from Mary and

Joseph (or the most loving woman and man you know) whatever you most needed at the moment of your conception.

✺ *Healing Actions for Oneself*

1. Visit a happily married couple. Before the visit, get in touch with whatever you most needed at the time of your conception. Go and enjoy the love between this couple.

2. Find a picture of your father, and put it in your pocket. Go for a long walk, imagining that you are your father's sperm on its way to meet your mother's egg. Notice what feelings and images come to you as you walk. Don't worry about getting it "right"—just trust what comes. Whatever comes, breathe the healing love of God into yourself and into your father.

3. Find a picture of your mother, and put it in your pocket. Find a safe and beautiful place in nature where you can sit and see a long way. Imagine that you are your mother's egg, waiting for the sperm that will become you. Notice what feelings and images come to you as you wait. Whatever comes, breathe the healing love of God into yourself and into your mother.

4. Plant seeds in a garden or indoor container. Care for them for the next nine months.

✺ *Healing Process for Unborn Children*

Parents can pray this for a baby with whom they are pregnant or for an older child.

1. You may wish to begin by lighting a candle and reading Luke 1:26–38.

2. Close your eyes and breathe deeply. One or both parents place their hands on the woman's body where the child was conceived. Count backward to the probable date of conception. Trust that there is a good reason for whatever date comes to you.

3. Imagine your child being conceived in this body. What was it like for your child to be a spirit merging with matter? To be merged with its father's sperm? To be merged with its mother's egg? To be merged with the relationship between its parents? What did your child most need?

4. Now breathe in from Mary and Joseph (or the most loving woman and man you know) whatever you imagine your child most needed at the moment of his or her conception. Breathe that out into your child.

✆ *Conception Game for Babies*

This game, which may be adapted for older children, recreates the experience of the sperm's head entering the egg. As your baby lies on his or her back, gently place your head on your baby's belly in a playful fashion. Then back away and notice any changes in the baby's breathing, the emotions in his or her eyes, level of bodily agitation, and so on. Repeat this a dozen times or so. Babies will often laugh or otherwise respond happily. But, underneath, you may notice subtle signs of agitation or a depth of feeling in the eyes. Empathically verbalize whatever you notice or intuit, by saying such things as, "Your eyes look sad," or "You're breathing faster—do you feel scared?" Then pick up the baby and lovingly comfort him or her.

Another version of this game, following the same guidelines as above for empathic verbalization and loving comfort, is to hold the baby upside down and gently place his or her head into the mother or father's belly, a bit like dipping a potato chip in some dip. Repeat this at about the same rate that you would dip potato chips in dip when you are hungry.

CHAPTER 5

❧

First Trimester: Physical Development

A normal pregnancy is approximately thirty-eight to forty-two weeks long. This time is commonly conceptualized as divided into three trimesters. The primary goal of the first trimester is physical development. In fact, by the end of the first trimester, all of the body's parts are developed, even though they must still mature. Trauma or stress interrupts the process of physical development and leaves long-term predispositions to illness. A general and widely accepted principle is that the impact of trauma during this period will be taken on by the physiological systems, body structures, and organs that are in a critical period of development when the trauma takes place.

For example, Dr. Graham Farrant, the world-renowned psychiatrist who, as mentioned earlier, helped pioneer research in cellular memory, was born with a disease involving the ventricle wall of his heart. During a regression to the prenatal period, he experienced his mother trying to abort him by alternating hot and cold baths. He sensed that this happened at exactly the most critical time for the development of the ventricle wall. He confronted his mother, who was astonished because she had never told anyone about the abortion attempt. She acknowledged that Graham's experience was correct. As the hurt of his mother's abortion attempt was healed, medically verified changes in Graham's heart occurred to the extent that he lived twenty years longer than medical experts expected. Not only the heart, as in Graham's case, but any bodily system can be impacted by trauma during the first trimester because all the systems are in critical stages of development during that time.

Any of us could tentatively guess when during the first three months of life we

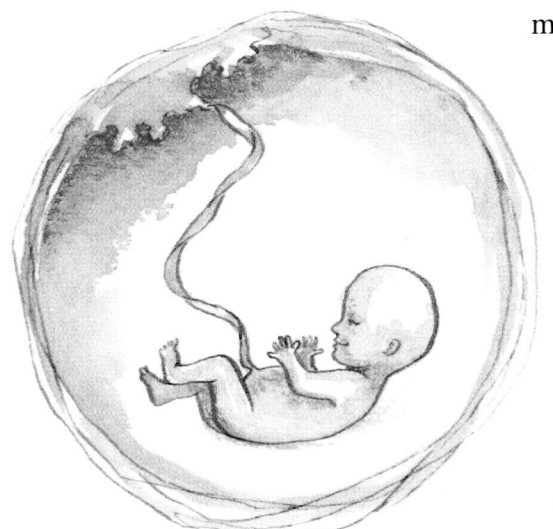

may have experienced trauma. First, we could notice which of our bodily systems are most prone to disease. We could then consult a chart of fetal growth (see Appendix) to find out when during the first trimester that system was in its critical period of development. Finally, we could seek healing of whatever trauma we might have experienced at that time. I (William) have seen many of my clients healed of physical illnesses in this way, including breast cancer, opthamological problems, and immune system disorders such as lupus. On the other hand, if we have a strong and healthy body, there is a good chance that our first trimester went well.

Implantation: More Deaths Occur in the Fallopian Tubes of Mothers Than at Any Other Place on the Planet

A critical event during the first trimester is implantation, the time when the baby implants into the uterine wall. The implantation journey, from conception through the fallopian tube to the uterine wall, involves the highest risk of complications and death than any other stage of life. The baby has seven days to implant for optimal chances of survival. Even one day earlier or one day later puts the baby at much greater risk.

In addition to a physical journey, a psychological journey is also taking place. Ideally, the psychological journey of implantation is experienced as finding one's home, a place to put down one's roots and belong. The gift of this journey in later life is the ability to find and make a home for oneself and for others.

Psalm 23, probably the most quoted of all the psalms, may have as one of its meanings the journey of implantation:

Yahweh is my shepherd, I lack nothing.
In meadows of green grass he makes me lie.
To the waters of repose he leads me;
there he revives my soul. . . .
Though I pass through a gloomy valley,
I fear no harm.

The uterine wall might be thought of as a garden in which the fetus searches for a place to grow—a "meadow of green grass" with "waters of repose," as the psalmist says. However, 50 to 75 percent of babies die during the period of implantation because they are not able to find a place in the uterine wall that is nourishing and supple enough to sustain life. Large areas may be unavailable because of fibroids, cysts, hardened tissue, and so on. Moreover, conscious or unconscious negative attitudes and feelings in the parents about conceiving a child or stress and trauma in their lives can make the ground of the garden hard and the soil poor.

Many life experiences may recapitulate trauma from the implantation journey. Every time we look for a home or even for a place to stay for the night, we may be recapitulating our implantation journey. The story of Joseph and Mary looking for a place to give birth to Jesus has many meanings, one of which may be as a metaphor for implantation. As Joseph and Mary searched for an inn where they could stay, rest, and go on toward birth, perhaps they were recapitulating their own implantations. When we imaginatively relive this experience with the Holy Family, we may be activating our implantation trauma and healing it.

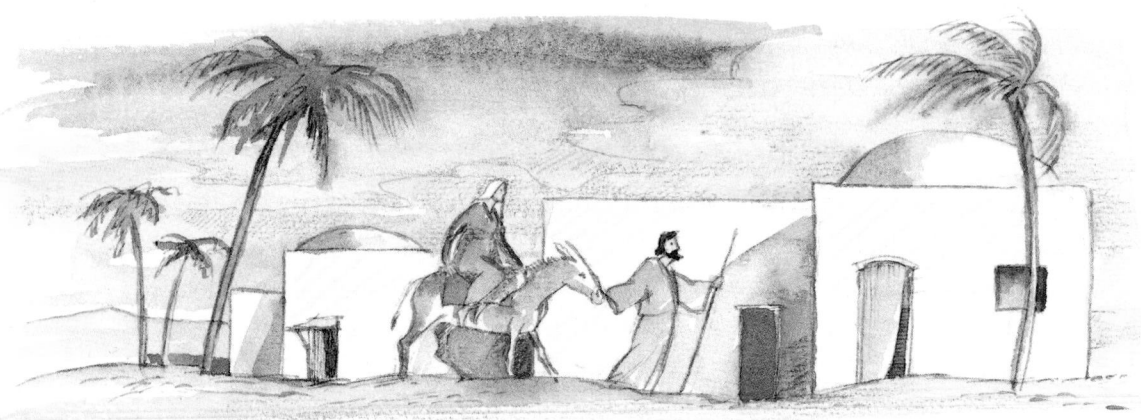

Discovery

After implantation, the next critical event during the first trimester is discovery. Discovery is the moment in every pregnancy when the mother first discovers that she is carrying a child. Ideally, this is a moment of celebration, in which the mother joyfully shares the good news with the father, the family, and friends. If joy and celebration are the prevailing attitudes of the parents when a child is discovered, for the rest of his or her life that child is likely to feel wanted and welcome in this world. He or she will feel confident of having a right to exist, take up space, be seen, and make an impact on the world.

However, if the parents are not happy to discover that they are pregnant, their child will have difficulty feeling wanted and welcome. Depending on the depth and duration of the parents' feelings of unhappiness and the extent to which their love is conditional (rather than unconditional), the child may struggle with issues ranging from shyness and insecurity to profound and crippling shame over his or her very existence. As an adult, he or she may find it hard to accept compliments and attention and may often feel like hiding. Often such a person, no matter how conscientious and successful, will feel like a fraud and fear being found out. Or, on the other hand, a person whose parents were not happy to discover him or her may compulsively seek compliments and attention throughout life without knowing why.

If the degree of rejection is extreme, the child may act out by repeating the parents' rejecting behavior. For example, four-year-old Mike continually kicked, hit, and pulled the hair of girls in his neighborhood. Mike's parents seemed to do everything right to help their son, but his behavior continued. Finally, in therapy he was regressed to the first trimester. He reexperienced his parents' intense fighting during this time regarding whether or not to abort him. Mike drew pictures of Mommy and Daddy "trying to kill each other." His parents acknowledged their discovery of him as the only time in their otherwise loving relationship when they had fought with each other.

In addition to fighting with other children, Mike was also very angry at God. He drew God as a big black hole. As he received treatment and resolved his feelings about his parents' fights, he no longer depicted God in negative ways. His behavior changed as well; he no longer attacked other children.

As in the example of Mike, the welcome babies receive in the first trimester affects their spiritual growth. If they are not welcomed in love, babies may reject the spiritual world in anger, as Mike did. My (William's) impression is that many agnostics and atheists had severe traumas during this time, and they unconsciously feel abandoned by a God whom they perceive as having done nothing for them. Or the response of a baby who experiences trauma may be the opposite of Mike's—he or she may want to leave his or her bodily existence and identify with the spiritual world only. In either spiritual response, the child may split off from himself or herself and lose firm contact with who he or she is at the deepest spiritual level.

Interaction of Physical and Emotional Factors

Although the first trimester is especially critical for physical development, this trimester illustrates the interplay of physical and emotional factors in human growth. On the one hand, emotional factors affect the formation of physical systems. For example, the time of discovery is also the time when the heart is developing. The human heart begins to beat three weeks after conception. This is the time when most women have missed their period for one week and are beginning to wonder if they might be pregnant. If the parents and their families rejoice in the pregnancy, the baby's entire system knows it, and the developing heart is likely to be strong.

However, if the pregnancy is unwanted, this rejection is passed on to the baby. The baby's cardiac system, which is in a critical period of development, will be most affected (as in the case of Graham Farrant). I (William) suspect that rejection at the time of discovery may be a major factor in the high incidence of heart disease in Western cultures, where one-half of all children are believed to be unwanted or ambivalently wanted.

While emotional factors affect physical development, physical factors also affect emotional development. An example is the effect of smoking, drugs, and alcohol during the earliest weeks of pregnancy, as described by Karr-Morse and Wiley:

> It appears that there is a period of great vulnerability to many types of drugs and to alcohol during the embryonic period, which is defined as the first eight weeks of pregnancy. This period, which precedes the period of fetal growth (eight weeks to delivery) is the time of *organogenesis*, when cells are first dividing, proliferating,

specializing, and then migrating to their permanent locations. Unfortunately, this is the time when many women are unaware that they are pregnant. . . . Many experts believe that fetal alcohol exposure, particularly because it may occur undetected and go untreated, may well be the single largest factor setting up physical and neurological conditions that predispose American babies to aggressive and violent behavior.

Thus, the effects of prenatal exposure to toxic substances can affect physical development—by damaging the nervous system and even altering genes—in such a way that healthy emotional growth may be disrupted.

Healing Attempted Abortion

The most traumatic experience a child can have during the first trimester (or at any other time during gestation) is attempted abortion. This is one of the deepest hurts possible and profoundly disrupts bonding between mother and child. An attempted abortion can result in lifelong, pervasive feelings of shame, fear of annihilation, and self-destructive impulses.

For example, Dr. Andrew Feldmar had some patients who had each attempted suicide five or more times at the same time each year. The dates seemed meaningless until Dr. Feldmar realized that each of these patients was attempting suicide at a time that would be the anniversary of his or her second or third month in the womb. When he investigated their histories, Dr. Feldmar discovered that the dates of the suicide attempts were the dates when each one's mother had attempted an abortion. Not only was the timing of each patient's suicide attempt reminiscent of an abortion attempt, but even the method was similar. One patient, whose mother had tried to abort him with a darning needle, tried suicide with a razor blade. Another, whose mother had used chemicals, tried suicide with a drug overdose. When Dr. Feldmar's patients realized that their suicidal ideas were really memories of their mothers' attempts to kill them, they were freed from the compulsion to commit suicide.

The depth of love required to heal abortion trauma is so great that—although we hesitate to make absolute statements—complete healing may only be possible through divine intervention. One source of divine intervention that we (Dennis,

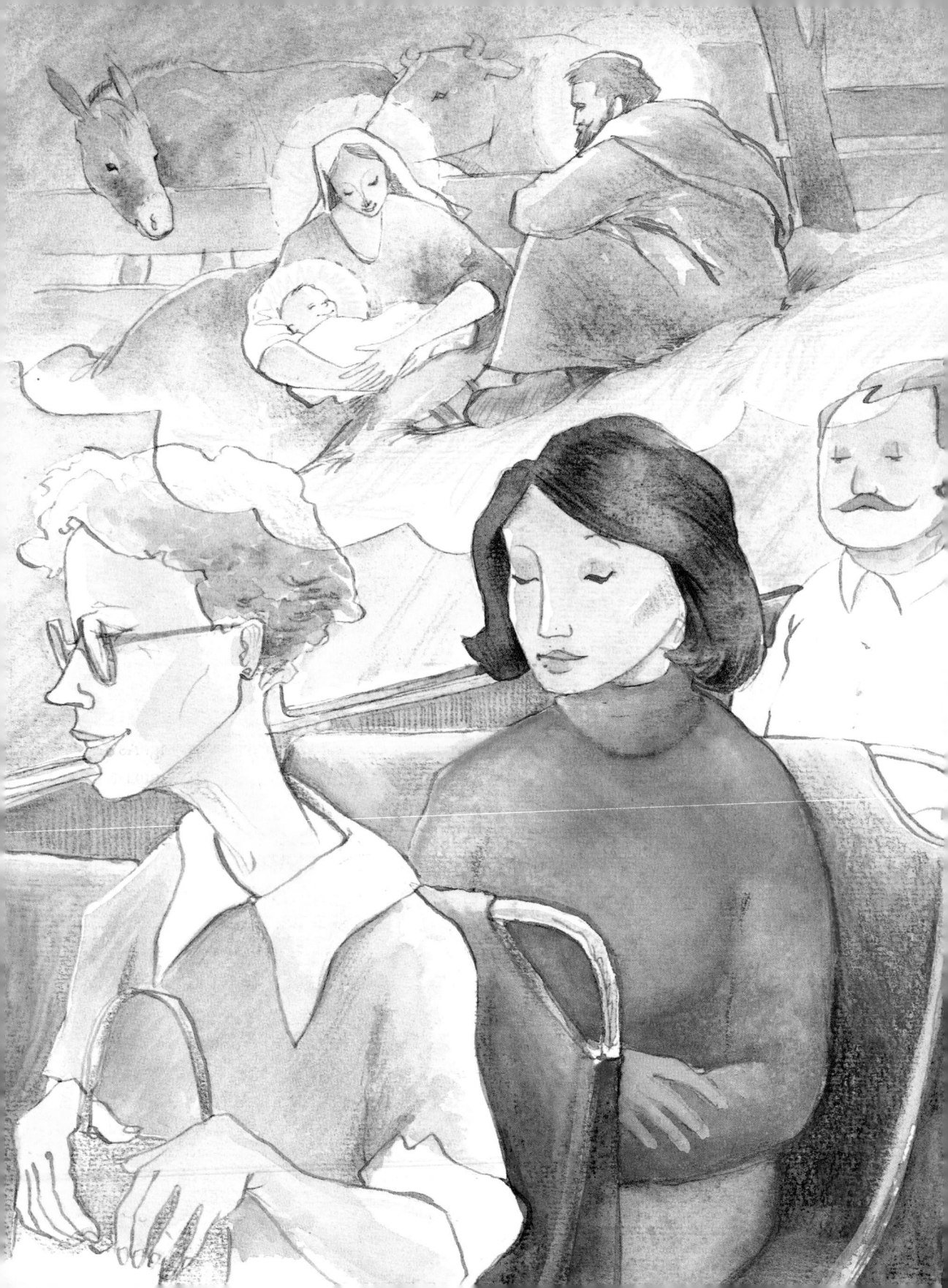

Sheila, and Matt) have found especially helpful with abortion trauma is the love of the Holy Family. For example, Mona had always felt distant from her mother, Ann, without knowing why. Ann was a loving, well-respected person, and Mona often berated herself for not feeling closer to her mother. One day, Mona was riding on a bus and reading the first chapter of our book, *Healing the Eight Stages of Life*. The chapter ends with a prayer inviting the reader to join Jesus at Bethlehem (similar to the prayer on pages 122–124 of this book). Although Mona was surrounded by noisy people, she felt drawn to do this prayer. She describes her experience as follows:

> I was summoned to use all of my senses to fully experience Bethlehem. So I did just that. I pictured Mother Mary, Joseph and Jesus in the manger, the animals surrounding them, and tried to hear the sounds that each animal would make. I also tried to feel the coldness of the night. When I tried to use my sense of smell, it became so evident that I actually smelled the manure of the animals around me. I suddenly felt God's presence and I was so grateful. As I was continuing to pray, I was asked to take Jesus' place and let Mary hold me in her arms. With this, I remarkably encountered Mary's loving arms around me and simultaneously felt the tremendous love of my own mother. I was in tears and I wanted to stay and feel that genuine love that I had never felt before.

Meanwhile, Mona's mother, Ann, was attending a conference on healing. As the entire group sang a hymn, one line from the song seemed to enter Ann's heart and lift the guilt that she had carried because she had tried to abort Mona. Ann decided to tell Mona about the abortion attempt and to ask her forgiveness. Now, Mona knew why she had felt distant from her mother all her life. Her experience on the bus had prepared her to appreciate how deeply her mother did love her, and Mona was easily able to forgive Ann. Mona began to feel so close to her mother that she decided to leave her job in a foreign country and move home so that their relationship could continue to grow.

Mona's story is notable not only for the depth of healing she experienced, but also because (like Dennis's need for breast-feeding described in Chapter 2) she didn't know at first what it was that needed to be healed. Like Mona, most of us don't consciously remember prenatal hurts. All Mona knew was that she wanted to be loved by Mary. The ways we most want to be loved are the ways in which we have been most hurt. Therefore, in a prayer experience such as entering the scene at

Bethlehem, we can trust that simply following our deepest desires to be loved will bring us the healing we need.

Moreover, usually we cannot fully face deep hurts until we have taken in love. In Mona's case, she took in Mother Mary's love, which opened her to Ann's love. Only then could she face the fact that her mother had tried to abort her.

Carried Feelings

What if Mona had not received healing for Ann's abortion attempt? If Mona herself someday became pregnant, she might feel ambivalent toward her baby without knowing why. As with so many prenatal and perinatal hurts, discovery trauma is often passed on unconsciously from one generation to the next.

For example, Dennis and Matt's sister Mary Ellen is adopted. Mary Ellen's birth mother did not want her. Consciously, Mary Ellen always wanted children. However, when she became pregnant, Mary Ellen was surprised to find herself apprehensive about being a mother. One day, she realized that these were not her own feelings— they were her birth mother's feelings, which Mary Ellen had absorbed and was now reliving. This awareness allowed Mary Ellen to let go of her birth mother's feelings and experience her own deep joy in being a mother. Her son David is now sixteen years old, and we have rarely seen a child as confident as he is of being wanted.

Like Mary Ellen, many people experience intense feelings that seem inconsistent with their conscious desires. Often these are "carried feelings," meaning that they belong to someone else and that we have picked them up from that person and are carrying them. This happens especially during the prenatal and perinatal period because the baby is so vulnerable to the feelings and attitudes of significant others and is unable to discriminate what feelings belong to whom. While she was pregnant with David, Mary Ellen was finally able to discriminate her own feelings about motherhood from those of her birth mother.

Even if we don't know whose feelings we are carrying, we can pray for healing. If we are aware of overwhelming feelings that seem inconsistent with who we are and what we want, we can give those feelings to God, asking God to carry them for the person to whom they belong. We can then ask God to fill in for us whatever we needed at the time we absorbed those feelings. We can also ask those who love us to give us what we still need.

We Need a Community to Delight in Us

One thing we all need is people who delight in us. For example, our (Dennis and Sheila's) John was hidden by his birth mother until she was nearly eight months pregnant. She was ambivalent about the pregnancy, and John's birth father had abandoned her. The birth mother was so isolated that she went to the hospital by herself in a taxi to deliver John at eight months and one week. We knew that John needed an intense experience of welcome, not only from us but from a large extended family and an even larger community of friends.

We sent a birth announcement to 500 people, inviting them to join us for John's baptism. Most sent cards and gifts, all of which we have saved to remind John that people all over the world rejoiced at his coming. Eighty of the people we invited traveled to our home to attend John's baptism, one from as far as the Philippines.

We believe that the core of baptism is delight in and welcome of a new member of the community. Baptism is well designed to heal discovery trauma, and we tried to take the fullest possible advantage of this. Thus, we asked each of our guests to bless John, one by one, with whatever most delighted them about him. For example, a person who noticed John's unusual focused attention blessed him with the gift of being present to others. Another person, knowing all John went through to be born, blessed him with the gift of overcoming obstacles.

When those eighty people blessed John with what delighted them about him, they were doing for John what empowered Jesus at his own baptism. When Jesus was baptized, he heard the words, "You are my beloved son in whom I am delighted." (Mk 1:11) Like Jesus and our son, to know that we belong in this world, we all need to experience that others delight in our coming. Perhaps it is no accident that the person Jesus chose to baptize him was John the Baptist, his cousin. The basis of Jesus' and John the Baptist's relationship was delight, beginning thirty years before when they were both in the womb and John leapt for joy at Jesus' coming (Lk 1:44).

☾ *Healing Process for Oneself*

This prayer is based upon the Visitation, when Elizabeth and the child in her womb, John the Baptist, delighted in Jesus. As a reminder that you are praying for a time when you were in an enclosed and darkened place, you may wish to do this

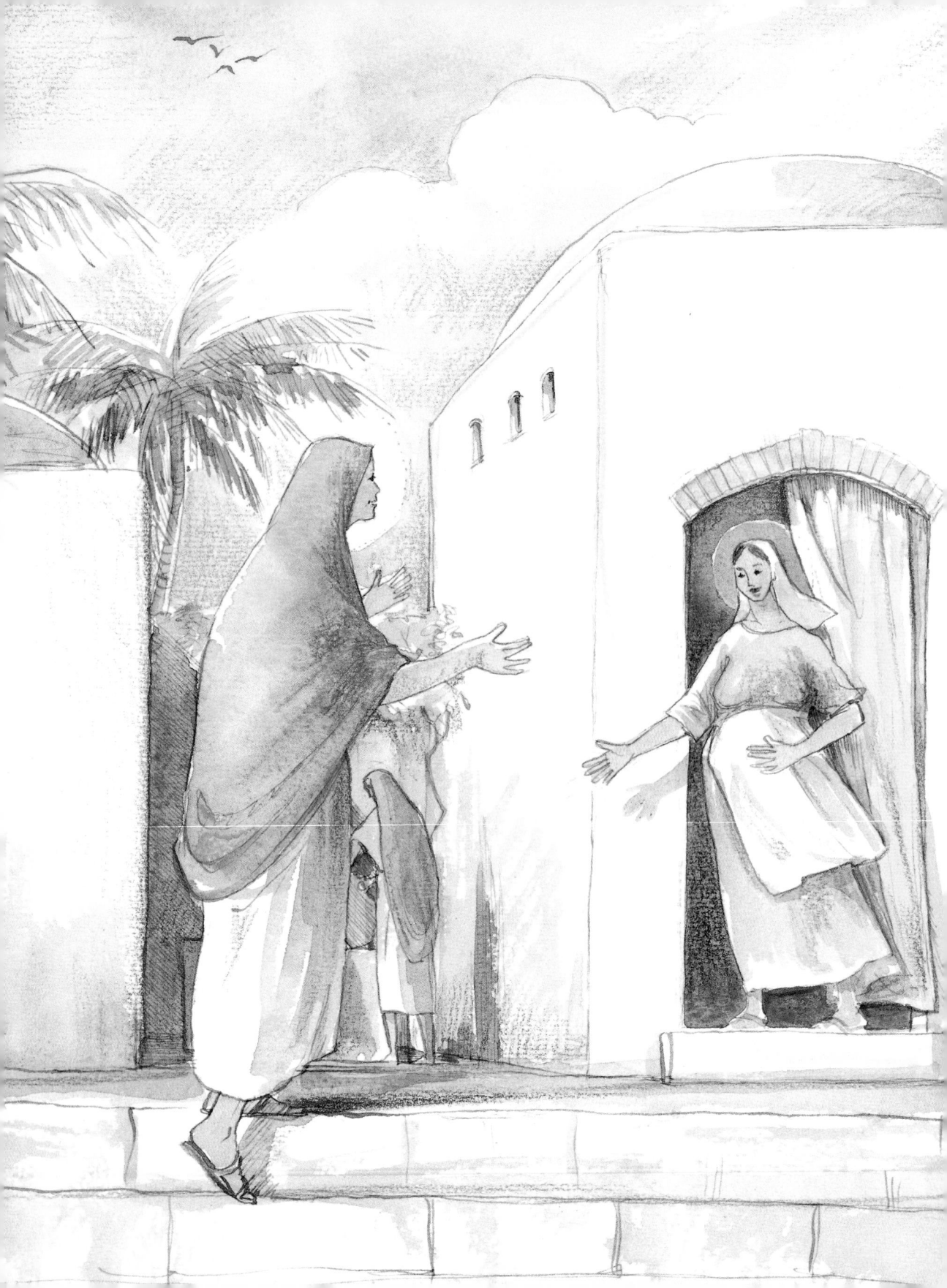

prayer in a closet, a small room with the door closed, or some other small, dark space. Notice which space feels exactly the right size for this stage of your development.

1. You may wish to begin by lighting a candle and reading Luke 1:39–56, the story of Mary's visit to Elizabeth.

2. Close your eyes and breathe deeply. Place your hand on your heart.

3. Imagine that you are being carried in your mother's womb under her heart. If your mother's womb was not a welcoming place, imagine that you are carried in the womb of Mary or of the most loving woman you know. Feel the warm fluid around you. Hear the heartbeat above you and the muffled sounds from the outer world.

4. Ask yourself whose delight in your coming would matter most to you. Invite those people to surround you as a baby in the womb. Perhaps you will also want to invite Mary's cousin (Elizabeth) and the baby in Elizabeth's womb (John the Baptist) to be present. Hear Elizabeth cry out to the woman who carries you, "The moment your greeting sounded in my ears, the baby leapt in my womb for joy." Let all the others whom you have invited express their joy over you and join Elizabeth and John the Baptist in blessing you.

5. Breathe in the love and welcome that surround you. Imagine it filling the moment when you actually were discovered. Let that love and welcome spread out through the entire first trimester of your life, touching any moments that may have been difficult. Breathe love into your body to heal the effects of alcohol, cigarettes, drugs, pollutants, or other toxic substances your mother may have ingested.

☙ *Healing Actions for Oneself*

1. Go to the place where you feel most at home. Ask yourself how you would like to change or add to this place, even in some very small way, so that you would feel even more at home. Do whatever comes to you.

2. Ask a friend whom you love and trust to look in your eyes and compliment you. Take in as many compliments as you can. If you reach a point where you are too uncomfortable to go on, ask your friend to stop. Repeat this process again a few days later, and see if you can take in more compliments this time.

❧ *Healing Process for Unborn Children*

During the first trimester of pregnancy, you may wish to pray for your child in the following way. Parents can also adapt this prayer for an older child.

1. You may wish to begin by lighting a candle and reading Luke 1:39–56.

2. Close your eyes and breathe deeply. One or both parents place their hands on the mother's womb. Based on what you know of your child's development at this stage, imagine how big your child is and how he looks.

3. Imagine Jesus, Mary, Joseph, and/or anyone else you trust placing their hands over yours. Breathe in their love for you and for your child. Breathe their love and yours out through your hands and into the child. Ask your child to tell you any hurts he may have experienced, including negative feelings you may have had about the pregnancy, thoughts of abortion, stress related to difficult circumstances in your own life, ingestion of toxic substances, and so on. Trust whatever comes to you, and ask that the love you are breathing into your child touch those hurts. Listen for any ways in which your child may want to communicate forgiveness to you.

4. Share with your child your delight in him, and listen for how your child may want to thank you for giving him life. Thank God for the gift of this child.

❧ *First Trimester Game*

Play Hide-and-Go-Seek with your child, showing great delight each time you discover each other.

CHAPTER 6

❧❧

Healing Twin Loss, Abortion, Miscarriage and Stillbirth

A deep hurt that often occurs during the first trimester (although it may happen at any time during the prenatal and perinatal period) is the loss of a child. In fact, many—perhaps most—of us have lost a brother or a sister. We say this because of the frequency of miscarriage, abortion, stillbirth, and twin loss. In the United States, approximately ~~15 to 20~~ 50 percent of pregnancies end in miscarriage, and there are about thirty-eight abortions for every hundred live births. Although the incidence of

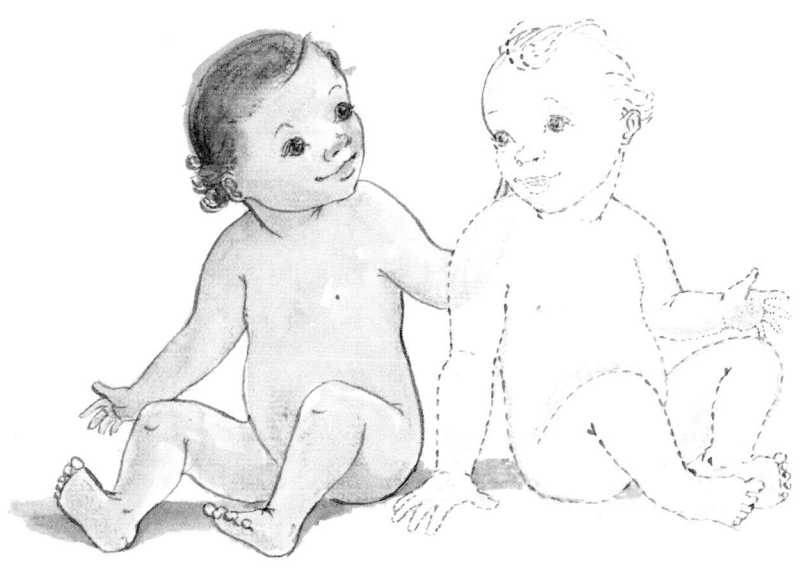

stillbirth has diminished greatly in recent years, at the time most of our readers were born, there were two stillbirths for every hundred live births. Embryologists estimate that 30 to 80 percent of us were conceived with a twin.

In Chapter 1, William described how profoundly the loss of his twin sister affected his life until he resolved that loss. In addition to twin loss, if our mother had a miscarriage, an abortion, or a stillbirth and that loss was unresolved, the effect on us can also be very great. We marinate in the unresolved grief of our parents, and we may have experienced our mother's womb as a burial ground, carrying the feeling and vibration of death. William calls this "the haunted womb syndrome."

Moreover, if parents have not grieved a lost baby, then they are unlikely to be emotionally available to fully bond with subsequent children. Just as in a broken marriage the previous spouse must be grieved before a healthy new marriage can be formed, so a lost child must be grieved before another child can be fully welcomed. If this doesn't happen, the next child is likely to suffer from diminished bonding with his or her parents.

Praying for Lost Babies

Children are very sensitive to the loss of siblings through miscarriage, abortion, or stillbirth, even when they have not been told about such losses. For example, Sue had six miscarriages before her daughter, Julie, was conceived. She had not grieved these miscarriages nor told Julie about them. Julie was emotionally fragile and cried easily. She had six dolls about whom she seemed to feel anxious and responsible. Each had a name, and each had to be accounted for at all times. After a retreat during which Sue prayed for healing of the loss of her miscarried babies, Julie's attachment to the dolls diminished. They became toys she played with but did not worry about. Her mother now describes her as more lively and happy and less emotionally fragile.

Another example is Sandy, who prayed for healing of her three traumatic miscarriages. She returned home to find her seven-year-old son, who had been hyperactive since birth, able to sleep through the whole night for the first time and to behave normally in school the next day. During the next weeks, her son's hyperactivity disappeared, as did his learning disabilities, which had been diagnosed as chronic and with a poor prognosis.

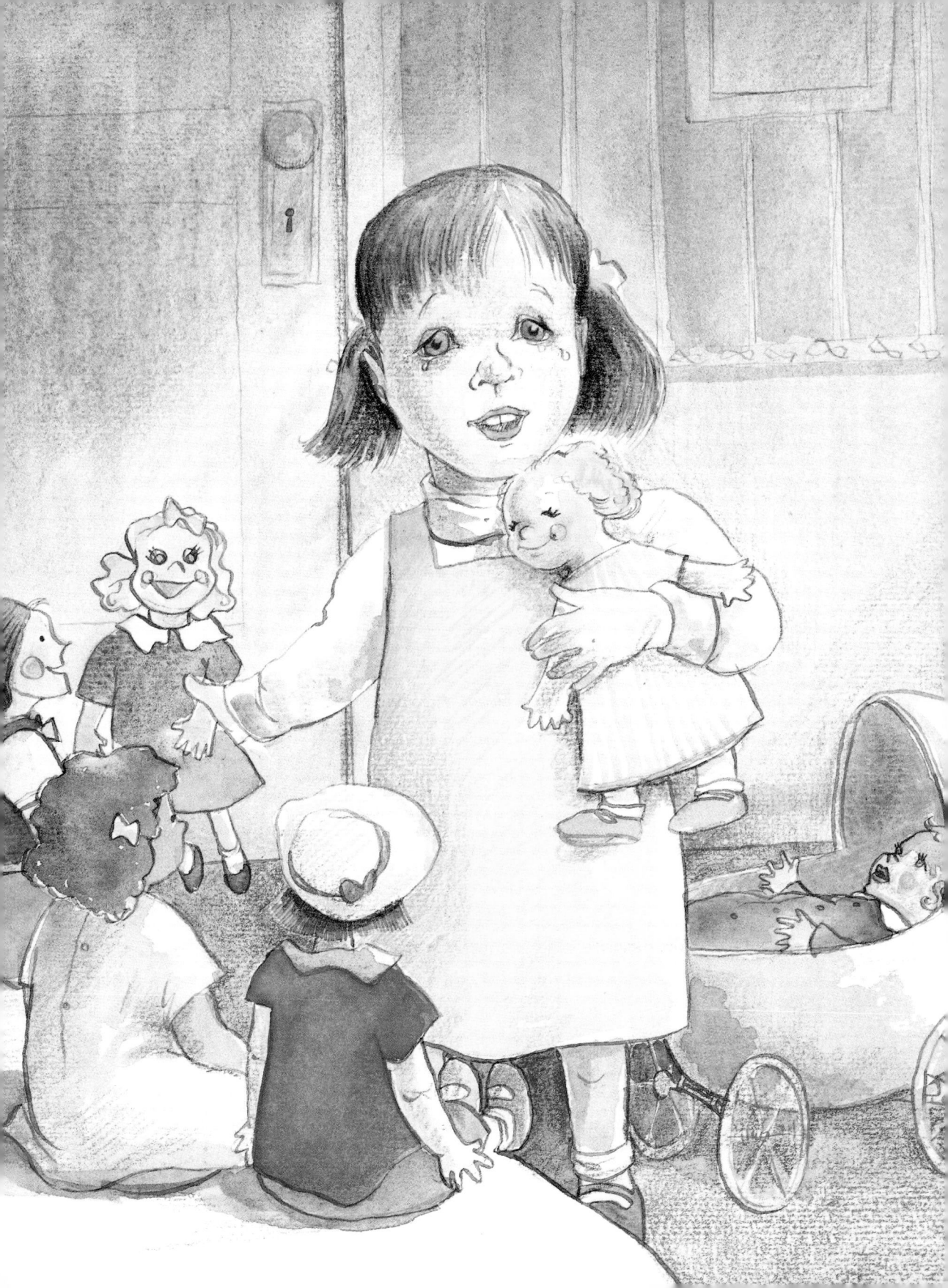

Just as the hurt of miscarriage can be healed, so can the hurt of abortion. Our friend, Char, told us the following story of one of her psychotherapy clients:

> I had been seeing Alice, age 38, for nearly a year for treatment of childhood sexual abuse. She told me of experiencing a sense of someone, a "being," following her around her home. "It feels like there is someone playing hide and seek. When I turn to look, I sense this 'someone' darting behind or into another room." She denied that she was frightened by this, but she felt "odd." Alice had never shown any evidence of distorted or altered thinking, so I did not think she was hallucinating or having delusions.
>
> I intuited that she might be dealing with a psychospiritual phenomenon related to an abortion. When I asked her if she ever had one, she admitted she had and that she had never told anyone about this.
>
> I suggested we do a prayer using guided imagery. I told her she would be in charge of the process and to let me know when she felt finished. I took her, through the use of her creative imagination, down a road to a stable where she met Mary, Joseph, and Jesus.
>
> I directed Alice to notice that Mary was holding a baby. The baby was Alice's. Mary offered the baby to Alice, who held him and talked with him. He assured Alice that he was safe and well cared for. Alice named him. After what seemed to her the right amount of time, I suggested to Alice that she return the baby to Mary's arms. She was relaxed and tearful.
>
> After this session, Alice reported that she was relieved of the sense that someone was following her. It was at this point in her treatment that the depression she had experienced began to lift. She began to have more energy to focus on the journey of healing sexual abuse.

We (Dennis, Sheila, and Matt) have prayed a similar prayer with thousands of women (and men) who, like Alice, have aborted a child. We have always been deeply moved by how quickly the child forgives the parents and how critical this forgiveness is for healing of the parents' guilt. Almost always, the child desires an ongoing relationship with the parents and their siblings. Often the aborted child seems to become an intercessor whose protective presence the family continues to sense.

Have You Lost a Child or a Sibling?

If you wonder whether you have lost a child or a sibling, you can ask the following questions. Because there could be many other explanations for "Yes" answers, they are only clues to the possible loss of a baby and not definite proof.

For Parents
- Mother: Did you experience any unexplained bleeding at a time when you were pregnant or could have conceived?
- Have you had cysts, tumors, fibroids, and/or other growths in your reproductive organs?*
- Mother or Father: Did you have repetitive dreams about loss during a time when the mother may have been pregnant?

For Siblings
- Did you have any imaginary playmates whom you insisted were real?
- Do you have repetitive dreams of someone you long for?
- Are your intimate relationships unsatisfactory, as if you are always searching for someone who does not exist? (This is sometimes acted out in the form of compulsive sexual behavior.)
- Do you have unexplained survivor's guilt (guilt about being alive while others die)?
- Do you have an unexplained fear of death (perhaps because a sibling died)?

☾ *Healing Process*

The following can be prayed for the loss of one's own child through miscarriage, abortion, or stillbirth. It can also be prayed for children who died shortly after birth.

---

*When miscarriages occur early in pregnancy, there is often an unconscious attempt to hold on to a lost child, even though the mother may be unaware of the loss. In several cases, tumors or cysts have been removed that contained hair follicles, bone cells, and other biological material from a miscarried child.

The healing that results can affect all the child's surviving brothers and sisters. This prayer can also be prayed by the one who has lost a sibling, such as a twin or from a pregnancy that occurred before or after one's own birth.

1. You may wish to begin by lighting a candle.

2. Close your eyes and breathe deeply. Recall a moment in your life when you knew how much God loves you. Breathe this love into yourself once again.

3. Get in touch with your feelings regarding the baby who died (love, sadness, longing, grief, guilt, anger, curiosity, etc.).

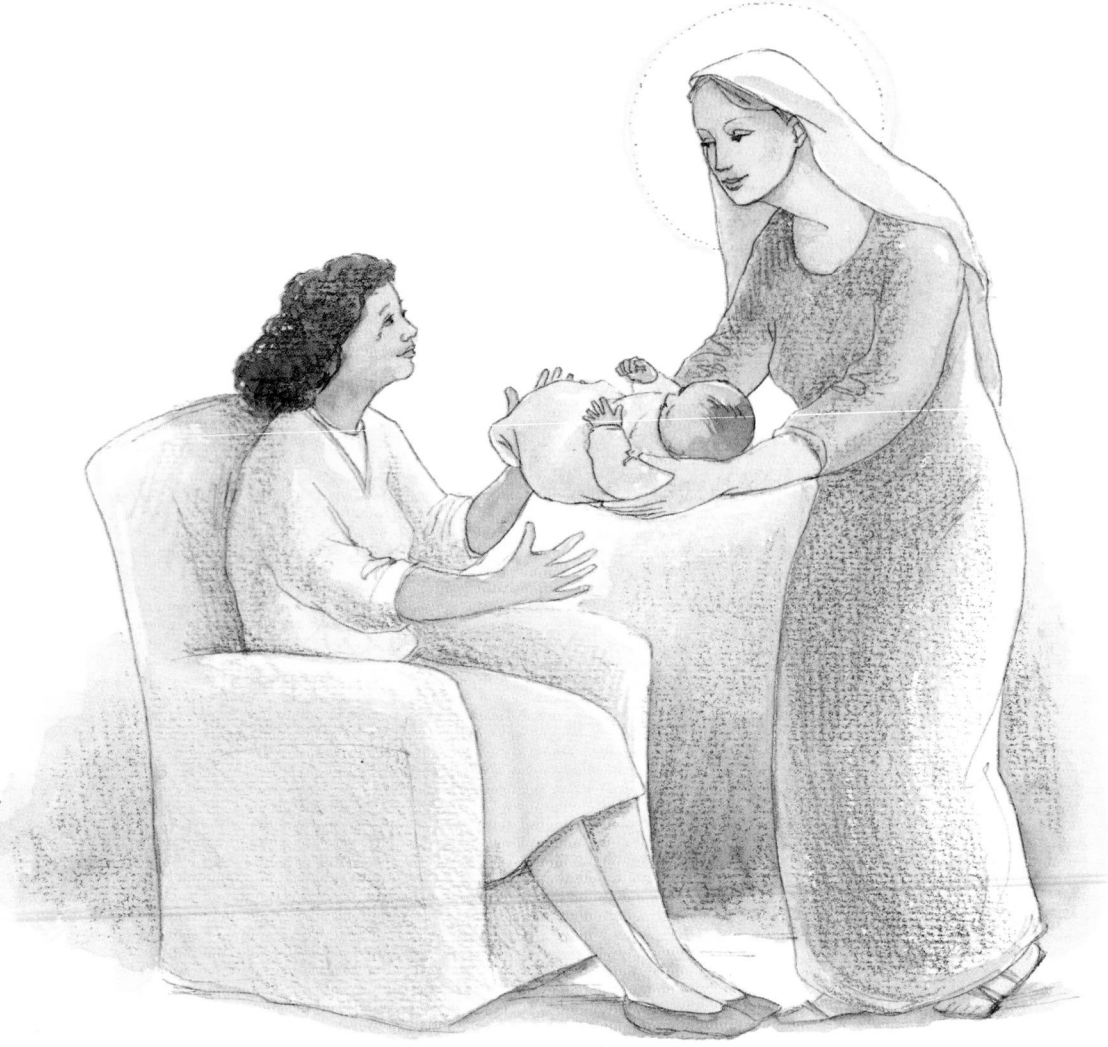

4. See Jesus, Mary, God the Mother, God the Father, or someone you love standing before you, holding your child or your sibling and offering him or her to you. Open your arms and receive the child. Say to and do with the child all that your heart has always longed to say or do, and let the child do the same for you.

5. See what sex the child is and ask what name he or she wishes to be called. If you are a Christian, you may wish to baptize the child. If so, make the sign of the cross on the child's forehead and say with Jesus, "I baptize you (name), in the name of the Father and of the Son and of the Holy Spirit." Imagine pouring water over the child's head, and feel the water cleansing and making all things new. If you are not a Christian, you may wish to bless the child in some other way consistent with your beliefs.

6. Talk over with the child how you can continue to give and receive love with each other. How do you want the child to pray for you and your family? How does the child want you to pray for him or her?

7. When you are ready, place the child in the arms of Jesus, Mary, or God. See that, instead of walking away from you, they walk *toward* you, right into your heart. Feel their warm presence as they make their home in your heart. Breathe deeply, allowing that warmth to fill your whole body.

✑ *Healing Actions for Oneself*

1. Go to one of your favorite places, where you feel most able to give and receive love. In your spirit, invite the lost child to accompany you. Share with him or her why this place means so much to you.

2. Ask yourself whom you would want as godparents for the lost child. Tell the child why you have chosen these people as godparents. Visit these people, and in your spirit bring the child with you. Invite the godparents to pray with you for the lost child and to bless him or her.

✆ *Game for Healing Loss of a Sibling*

If you know that your child has lost one or more siblings, find a time when you feel especially connected to your child. Create as safe and warm an environment as possible, in which your child's favorite dolls or stuffed animals are nearby. Tell your child as much as you know about the loss. Ask your child if any of the dolls or stuffed animals have anything they want to say, or if he or she wants to say anything to or do anything with the dolls or stuffed animals. Follow the child's lead, and mirror back to the child any feelings he or she expresses. Talk over with the child what name to give the lost sibling. During the next days and weeks, offer the child additional opportunities to express any feelings about the loss with the help of the dolls or stuffed animals.

CHAPTER 7

Second Trimester: Spiritual Development

If you want to try an experiment, go outside on a star-filled night and lie down in a safe place. Consciously release any tension you may be carrying from the day. Open yourself to the enormity, the beauty, and the mystery of the universe. As you do so, notice if any tension recurs or even increases in your body. There should be little or none because you are so close to the universe. If there is any tension, this may reflect your resistance to connection to forces greater than yourself, and it may mean that you were wounded during the second trimester.

The main developmental task of the first trimester is physical growth. By the end of the first trimester, all the parts of the body are present in elemental form and only need to mature. The main task of the second trimester is the development of the spiritual aspects of the inner self (the psychological aspects of the inner self will develop in the third trimester).

The second trimester is a time of quiescence, a time for the soul to rest before the advent of the ego (which develops primarily during the third trimester, if there have been no traumas). It seems significant that it is during the second trimester that many pregnant women feel their best physically and thus most able to provide a restful environment for their babies.

Most spiritual traditions recognize that quietness of body and mind leads to inner spiritual experience. This is precisely what occurs during the second trimester: the body is developed sufficiently to no longer be the focus of attention, and the mind is still quiet. The baby meets the Holy Spirit, the Christ Child, and God as Mother and Father in a "bodily-felt way." The second trimester baby also experi-

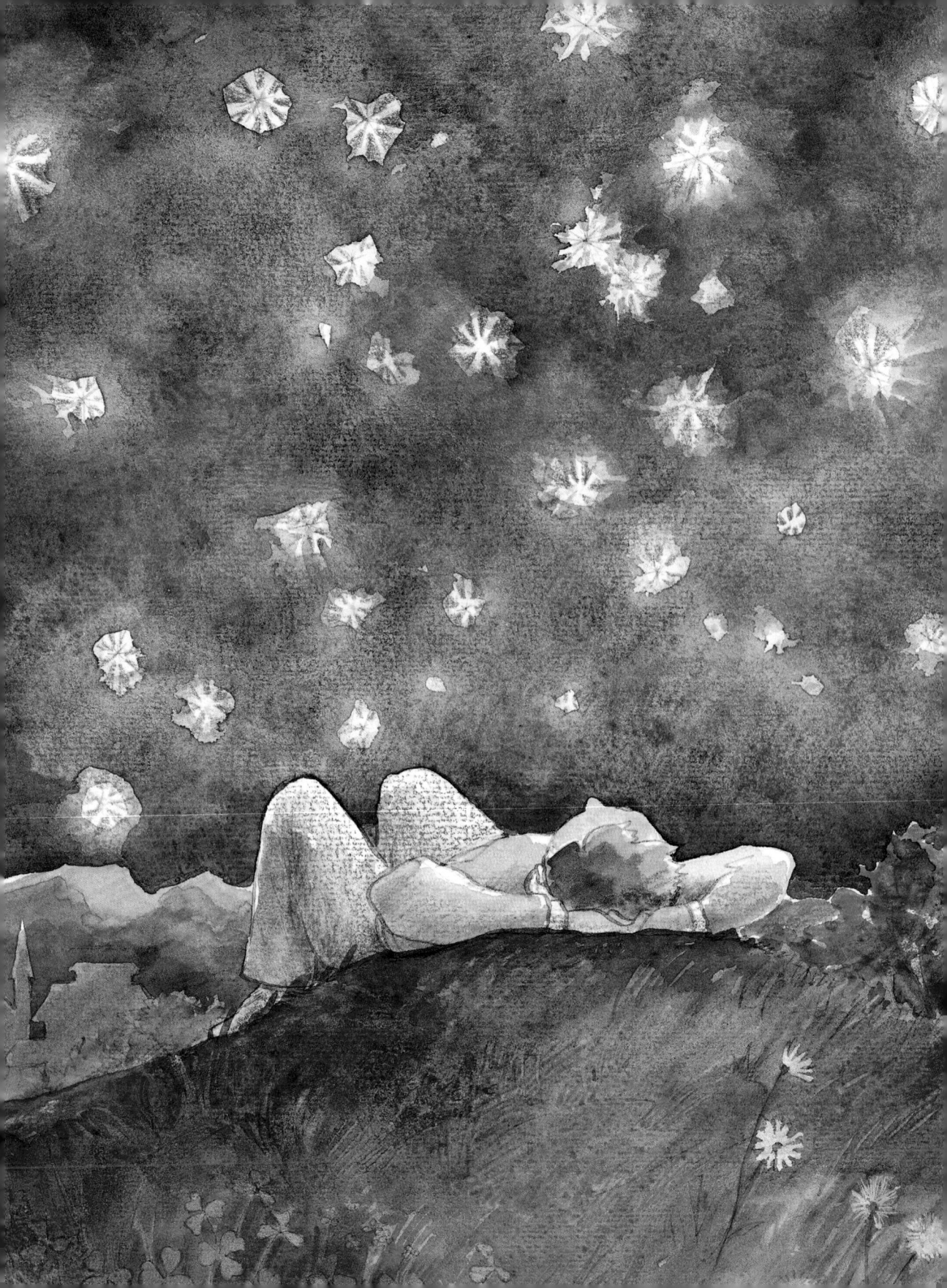

ences a natural capacity for loving union that spiritual seekers may spend a lifetime trying to recover. As theologian Daniel O'Hanlon writes,

> . . . It is possible to allow love to simply emerge out of awareness, without making its cultivation the first object of concern. . . . Love and compassion are the natural movement of our true self. When the surface mind and disordered desires are still, the true self awakens without need of any further assistance from us. Indeed, our clumsy efforts to poke at it and deliberately rouse it often have the same effect as poking at a sea anemone. It simply closes up tight. But give it stillness, leave it undisturbed, and it opens wide like a water lily in full bloom.

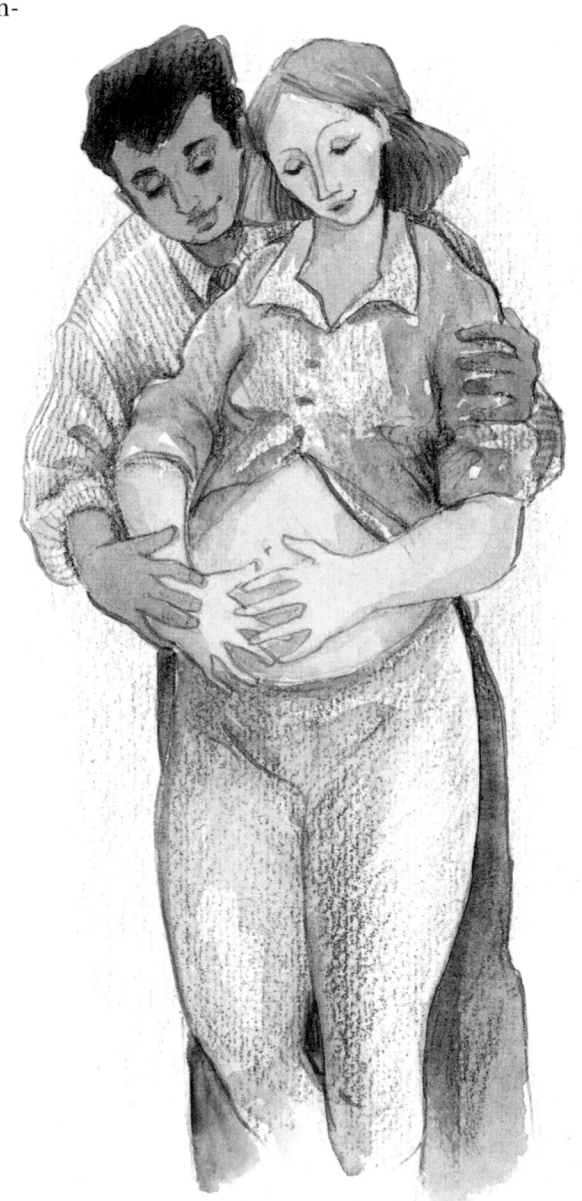

A healthy second trimester baby is "opening wide like a water lily in full bloom."

During these months, for the first time, the prenate comes to terms with his or her spiritual self in the form of imagination, creativity, intuition, awareness, and, most of all, spiritual experiences. It is normal for the baby's inner self to roam freely, to experience God in the form of spontaneous reverie, images, symbols, sounds, and energies. When adults are regressed to the second trimester, they report encounters with the spiritual ground of their being.

Hurts During the Second Trimester

Because second trimester babies are so exquisitely spiritually sensitive, it is the capacity for spirituality that is most damaged by trauma during this time. The trauma then becomes an associational link, so that every time an attempt is made to connect with one's inner life or with God, the unresolved traumas are also unconsciously reactivated. This brings turmoil into the spiritual process. This turmoil may be expressed in either of two ways: by an aversion to spirituality, or by a fixation on one narrow form of spirituality.

For example, a child with whom I (William) worked had an aversion to God. When I asked him what he had against God, he said, "Every time I think of God, I get a headache." When I asked him to go to any experience in his life that would help him understand this feeling, he regressed spontaneously to the second trimester. Here he found his answer. His sister, who was three years old when he was a second trimester prenate, became very ill. His distraught parents virtually forgot about him for a period of time. This event interrupted his natural process of connection to God. He began to associate God and spirituality with the abandonment and fear he experienced from his parents. Thus, he developed an aversion to God.

On the other hand, second trimester trauma can cause a person to become fixated in a particular spiritual mode. There are many aspects of God and ways of relating to God, and during the second trimester these are all accessible to the prenate.

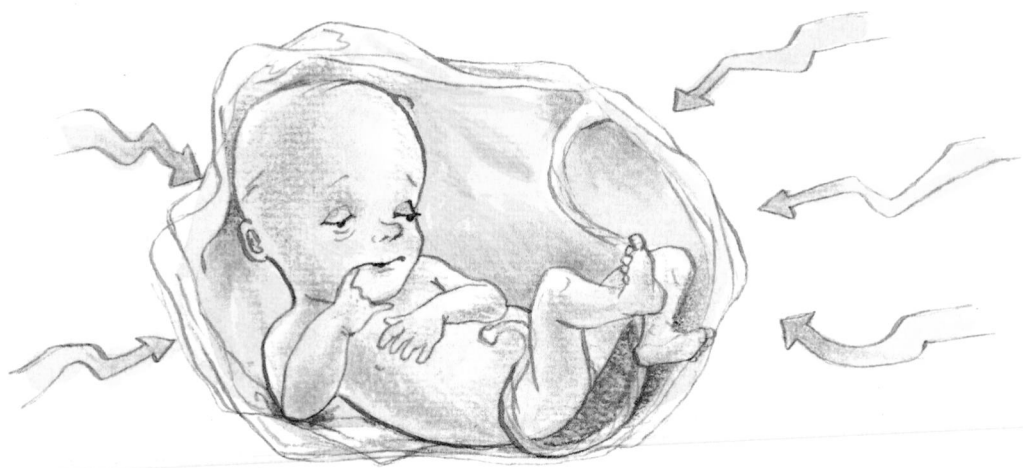

However, if the prenate experiences trauma, he or she may latch onto only one way of relating to God. In other words, the prenate desperately mobilizes a particular spiritual mode for survival, as a defense. This may be expressed in adulthood through the insistence that the Bible or the rosary or the Eucharist or vegetarianism or serving the poor, and so on is the *only* way to God.

Whether a person has a fixation on one particular form of spirituality or an aversion to all forms of spirituality, spiritual experiences later in life can trigger the recovery of trauma memories. A second trimester baby may see mandalas, hear voices, see lights, have visions, or simply feel God's presence. As an adult, seeing a mandala, having a vision, feeling God's presence, and so on may trigger feelings of terror, rage, and the like. Some might interpret this as an "attack" by evil spirits, when in fact it may simply be a need for healing during the second trimester.

What we have just said about spiritual experiences also relates to "inner work." A second trimester baby is in touch with his or her inner self. If that baby is traumatized, trying to contact the inner self as an adult through such processes as journaling, creative imagination, and deep breathing, may trigger intense distress. Such activities require stillness, and stillness itself may trigger distress if the quiescence of the second trimester was disrupted by distressing events.

Trauma Includes More Than the Parents

Throughout the prenatal and perinatal period, babies can be traumatized not only by the difficulties of their parents, but also by many factors in the environment. This includes medical interventions such as sonograms, amniocentesis, and other invasive procedures. For example, Dr. David Chamberlain writes:

> Researchers have observed a strange response to withdrawal of amniotic fluid after amniocentesis. In this procedure, which has become increasingly common, a needle penetrates the womb to withdraw a sample of fluid to verify possible genetic defects. Prenates about sixteen weeks from conception were filmed after needle puncture by doctors in Denmark. Half of them showed a striking, somewhat ominous reaction: they didn't move for two minutes.
>
> Half of them also lost the variations normally found in a series of heartbeats. This flat, unvarying heartbeat pattern is also seen in very sick babies or babies who

have been hit by a dose of Valium or some other drug. Because none of the fetuses showed this pattern before amniocentesis, researchers conclude they were reacting to the procedure itself. What we see here is not indifference, but a sensitive, perhaps shocked reaction to what has just happened in the sanctuary where they live.

As in the above example, second trimester babies are acutely conscious, sensitive, and responsive to the world around them.

Relating to a Second Trimester Baby

My wife and I (William) experienced the sensitivity and responsiveness of our son, Jamie, during a prenatal medical procedure. The doctors told us they needed to do some ultrasonic screening. Although we knew that this procedure was invasive, the circumstances were such that it seemed necessary. To minimize the trauma, we prepared Jamie by explaining to him what would happen and why it was necessary.

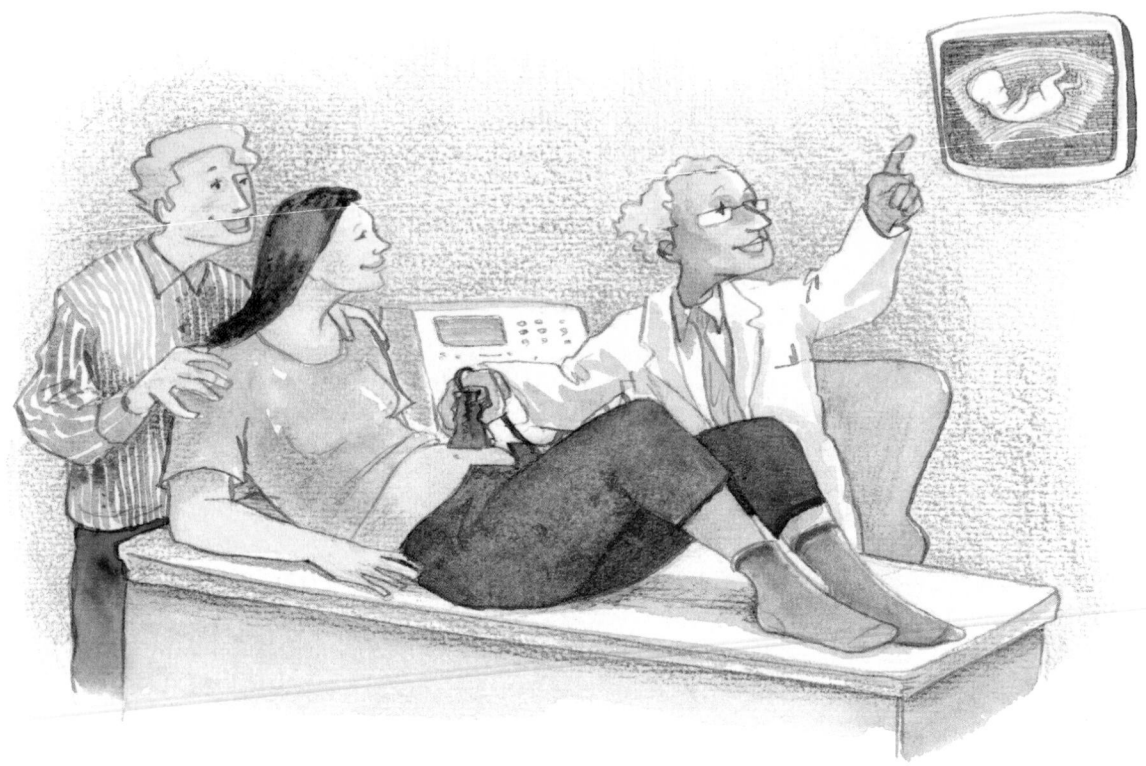

During the sonographic imaging, as our son appeared on the screen, I asked the doctor and the nurse if they thought babies at this stage were aware of what was happening to them. They both gave me a strange look and said something like, "Of course not!" I noticed that Jamie was curled up on the bottom of the womb, unlike his usual lively self. The doctor and the nurse then left the room briefly. As soon as the door closed behind them, Jamie jumped up, did three somersaults, and moved his hands as if waving to us. The doctor and the nurse returned, and immediately Jamie curled up on the bottom of the womb once more. I believe babies know when their awareness and their capacity for relationship are respected and when they aren't.

One person who understands this is Dr. Franz Veldman, a Dutch scientist who developed "haptonomy," the science of touch. He teaches parents to make loving contact with their unborn child beginning in the second trimester. Dr. Veldman asks the parents to place their hands on the womb and to get in touch with all their love for their child. If they focus their love especially through the hands on the right side of the womb, the child will begin to move to that side and curl up with his or her neck under those hands. If they then focus their love through the hands on the left side of the womb, the child will move to that side and curl up under those hands. In this way, the parents can rock the child back and forth. If they do this at the same time each day and then miss their "visit" with the child one day, the child will begin to kick, as if in protest.

Second trimester babies relate not only through touch, but in many other ways, such as through sound. As far back as 1955, Dr. Henry Truby analyzed infant cries to produce "cryprints," detailed sound portraits as unique to babies as their finger-prints:

> In the cryprints of premature infants five months old, weighing only nine hundred grams, they found a correspondence to intonations, rhythms, and other speech performance features of the mother. This revolutionary discovery meant not only that the infants were hearing their mothers but had been taking language lessons. The unborn babies had already acquired some of their mothers' personal accents and speech sounds.

The baby's response to sound is discernible to the mother. For example, a study in a London hospital found that by four or five months in the womb, babies respond

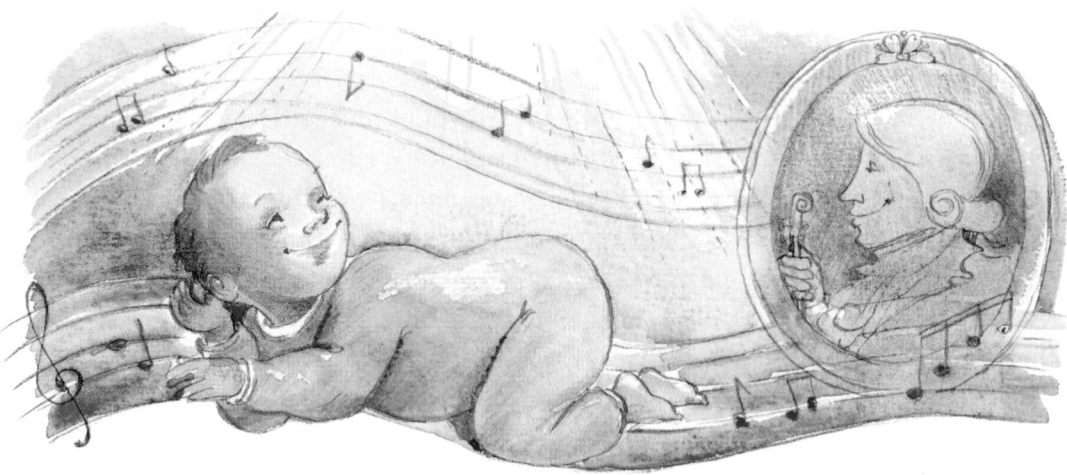

consistently to various types of music. They grow calm in response to Vivaldi and Mozart, whereas they become restless (indicated by kicking, etc.) in response to Beethoven, Brahms, and hard-rock music. This sensitivity to music is another indication of spiritual development because music has long been recognized as a way of opening one's spirit.

Creating a Loving Environment

During the second trimester, perhaps the greatest hurt is to be surrounded by parents and a culture that denigrate spirituality. A great gift to a child during this time is to be in an environment that fosters spirituality. Maybe this is why, in traditional Jewish culture, a pregnant woman would leave her husband and her other responsibilities and go to the home of a friend or a relative who could provide care and seclusion. During her time away, she would pray, ponder the scriptures, and focus her thoughts on God to give her child a beautifully formed soul. Mary followed this custom when she visited her cousin, Elizabeth, for three months.

Mary and Elizabeth gave and received affirming love with each other, and this affected the babies in their wombs. In Native American culture, there is a similar custom: a pregnant woman goes off with loving female friends who care for her and braid her hair. These customs reflect an understanding that the expectant mother needs to be mothered (and, we believe, the expectant father needs to be fathered).

During the second trimester of our John's prenatal life, no one cared for his birth mother. No one else even knew that she was pregnant. Moreover, she did several things that could have been very harmful to John, such as smoking regularly, drinking alcohol, and living on the streets in the midst of violence. Although we (Dennis and Sheila) were not biologically pregnant, we were already carrying John in our hearts during this time. Fortunately, we were surrounded by a loving community that cared for us and John just as Elizabeth cared for Mary and Jesus.

One member of our community is Char. After John was born, she shared with us the following entry from her journal, written during John's second trimester:

> It's been several years since the compelling body-felt desire to have children was laid to rest within me. So, why am I experiencing this tremendous urgency and longing to bear and nurture the development of a baby? Why this internal cry of the womb reverberating with every heartbeat, "I can hold, I can carry, I can feed . . . I am holding, I am carrying, I am feeding!?"
>
> Perhaps I really can hold, carry and feed! I wonder, is this the way in which I'm being called to pray for Dennis and Sheila? Do they need someone to hold their baby for a while? Perhaps, my body could carry the prayer that my heart is holding! How awesome, how very possible. I could do this. I will do this! I will carry their baby if that's what they need.
>
> Even as I ponder the possibility, I sense my womb swelling with the warmth of a living presence! I walk with a deep body-felt sense that I am already incubating and nurturing the life I hold in my heart's prayer for Sheila and Dennis! This is incredible, and I must be careful to share this discriminately with friends who can lovingly advise me.
>
> So, I prepared myself psychologically to be a surrogate mother . . . to hold and nurture the child of Sheila and Dennis. I did not share my experience with them at the time, because I needed to consult with a professional expert. When I did, I discovered that fibroids lining my uterus, which had been treated in the past, had grown back. The chances of a baby's body nesting were too slim. I was disappointed, and the best way I could explain the experience of my body was that my prayer had become concretized in the womb. I planned to share this with Dennis and Sheila at an appropriate time after the arrival of their baby.

Although Char knew nothing of John until after he was born, her experience was most intense during his second trimester. This was exactly the time when his birth

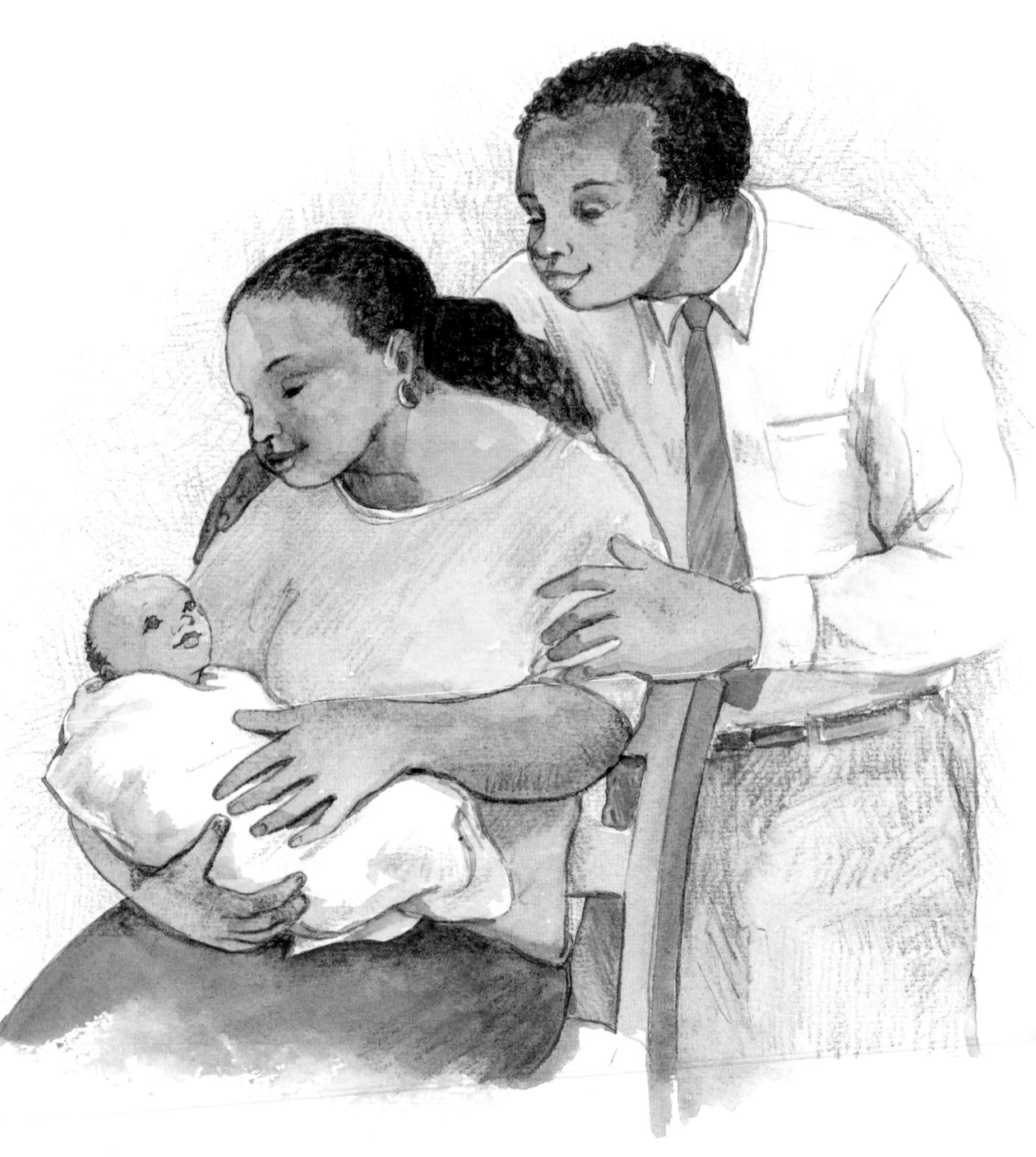

mother's behavior was most potentially dangerous to him. Char mistakenly thought that the reason we had not conceived was that Sheila could not carry a baby; however, she rightly intuited John's need for a safe womb.

When I (William) first examined John at three weeks of age, given his prenatal history I expected him to have very serious symptoms. In fact, he had only about 20 percent of the trauma that I would have predicted, and it was evident to me that this trauma could easily be resolved. I believe John was protected by the love and prayer of Dennis and Sheila, his Uncle Matt, and members of their community, like Char.

We all believe that John's extraordinarily good physical and emotional health comes from the fact that, in a certain sense, he spent his second trimester in two safe wombs (Sheila's and Char's). This protected him from the lack of safety in his birth mother's womb. Often when we have prayed with a person whose birth mother's womb was unsafe, we have placed that person in the womb of Mary, who can fill in what that person needed. We pray this way for John every night.

☾ *Healing Process for Oneself*

The following prayer is based on the Jewish custom in which a pregnant woman goes to a safe and loving place where she can be cared for, as Mary did when she visited Elizabeth.

1. You may wish to light a candle. Close your eyes and breathe deeply.

2. Imagine that you are in your second trimester of life in the womb. Ask yourself where your mother would have been most safe and loved as she waited for your birth. Perhaps you will think of your grandparents' home, perhaps the home of another family member or of your parents' closest friends, perhaps their church or other faith community, perhaps a favorite family vacation place. If you cannot think of any safe place that was available to your mother, imagine a place where you wish she could have gone, such as the home of Mary and Joseph or the home of Mary's cousin, Elizabeth.

3. Now imagine your mother, perhaps accompanied by your father, going to this place. Hear the loving voices that surround your mother, and feel the gentle ways

in which people touch the outside of her womb, hoping to feel your tiny body. Breathe in the ways God is caring for your mother through her friends and family, as their love fills your mother and is transmitted to you across the placenta.

4. If you know of any way in which you were hurt during your second trimester, breathe healing love especially into those hurts.

☞ Healing Actions for Oneself

1. Find a safe, warm, clean place that smells good. Bring with you a cassette tape player and a favorite blanket. Wrap yourself in the blanket, and listen to a tape of music by Mozart, Vivaldi, or your favorite composer. You may instead wish to play "Transitions," a series of tapes of womb sounds combined with beautiful music. (Available from Transitions Music, P.O. Box 8532, Atlanta, GA 30306; 1-800-492-9885.)

2. At another time, you may wish to ask a person whom you love and trust to help you with the above. Begin in the same way, and then ask that person to put his or her arms around the outside of the blanket and rock you back and forth, or stroke the blanket gently but firmly enough for you to feel his or her care, as you continue listening to the music.

☞ Healing Process for Unborn Children

1. Close your eyes and breathe deeply, centering yourself in the love of God and breathing that love into the child you are expecting.

2. Ask yourself and your child where would be the safest and most loving place you could go, where both of you (or all three of you, if the father is sharing in this prayer) would feel loved and cared for.

3. If possible go to that place, even for a short visit. If you cannot go there physically at this time, go there in your imagination. While you are there, consciously take in love and care for yourself and for your child.

☾ *Second Trimester Game*

You may wish to play this game with a child who is old enough to speak. Find a time when several family members or friends are available to help.

Form a circle around the child and the mother. Ask the child to imagine being a baby in the womb. Ask the child how close or how far away the circle of people should be. Ask the child if she would like the people to sing a song of love and welcome and what that song should be. Ask the child if there is anything else she wants the people to do. If the child has no requests, the group members can express to the child how much they love and appreciate her.

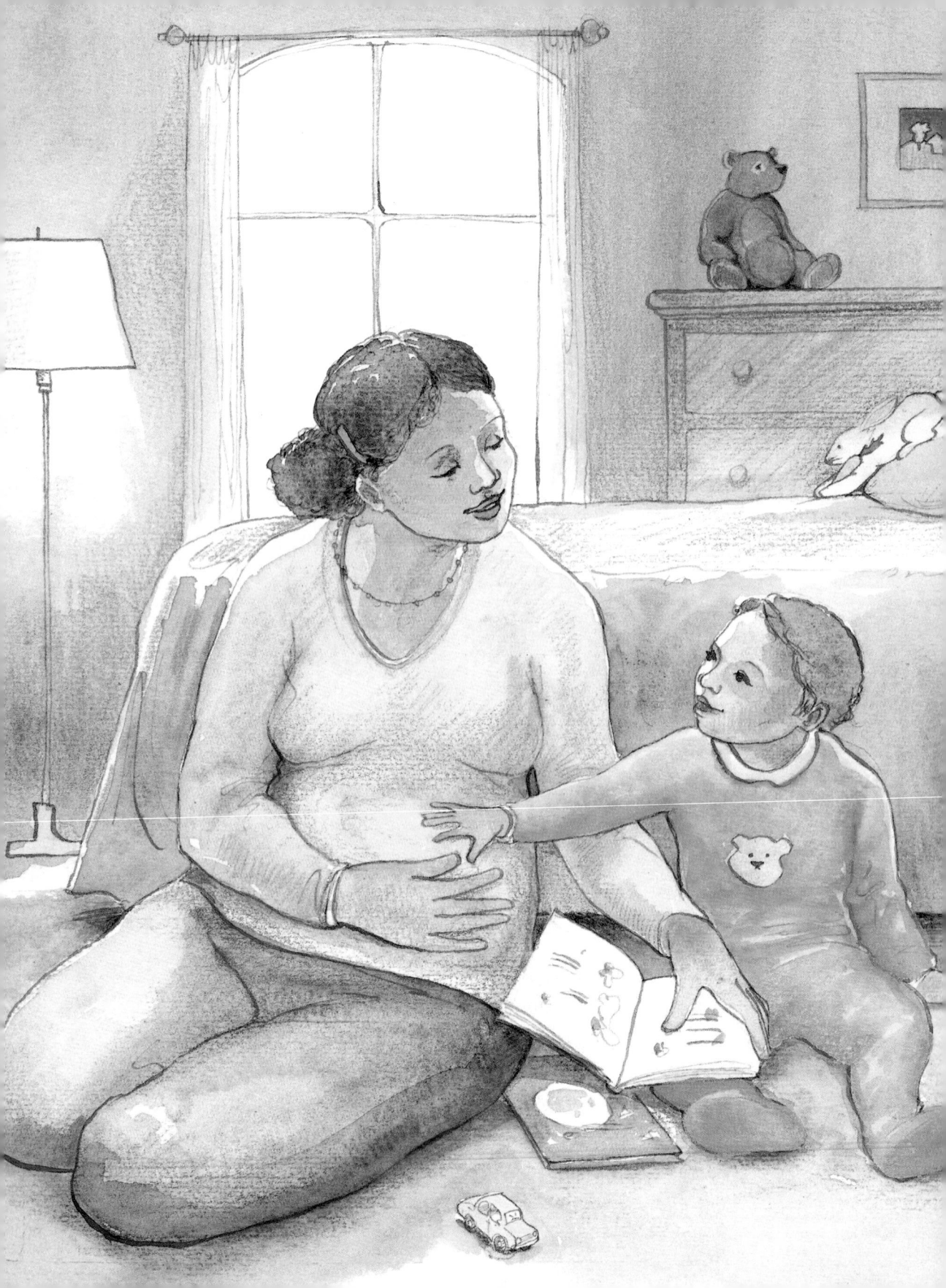

CHAPTER 8

❦

Third Trimester:
The Individuating Self

Dr. David Chamberlain reports an experiment in which every member of a group of twenty-six expectant mothers correctly identified the sex of their baby prior to a sonogram or birth. Dr. Beatriz Manrique reports a similar experiment devised by a group of fathers attending her Hello Baby childbirth classes in Venezuela (mentioned in Chapter 1). The fathers wondered whether their baby would be a boy or a girl but were too poor to arrange for sonograms. They devised the following experiment. Each father told the baby in the mother's womb to kick once if she was a girl and twice if he was a boy. The next week in class they made a list of their answers. After the babies were born, Dr. Manrique checked the list. All ten fathers were right.

Hello Baby includes exercises for prenates developed by Dr. Rene Van de Carr at his Prenatal University program in Hayward, California. One of Dr. Van de Carr's exercises is the "Kick Game." Beginning in the fifth month of pregnancy and continuing through the third trimester, when the baby starts to make kicking motions, the parents can gently press where the baby kicked while saying, "Kick, kick." Eventually, the baby may start to kick back. In some cases, once communication is established, each time the parents vary the number of presses, the baby will respond with a similar number of kicks.

In another of Dr. Van de Carr's exercises, also beginning in the fifth month, the parents repeat a list of words including *pat, rub, squeeze, shake, stroke,* and *tap*. The baby not only hears each word but at the same time feels the parents doing each of these actions on the mother's womb. One mother, now five months pregnant, had done this when she was pregnant with her daughter, now sixteen months old. She had never told her daughter about this. One day mother and daughter were sitting on the floor and the mother said, "Look at mom's big tummy; mommy has a baby in

will have a profound impact on the child. In fact, when parents feel stress, prenates feel even more stress because they are so powerless and have so little defense.

Parents experience many stresses during the last months of pregnancy. These may include changing or quitting jobs to be with the baby, taking on new jobs to make more money to support the baby or buy a larger home, etc. Mothers may be increasingly uncomfortable physically, and first-time parents especially may feel anxiety about childbirth. Because whatever is stressful for mothers is geometrically more stressful for babies, this can predispose the baby to anticipatory anxiety later in life in any situation that symbolizes birth. Thus, life transitions such as college entrance exams, interviewing for a job, and getting married can be colored by the mother's anxiety about birth that permeated into the child.

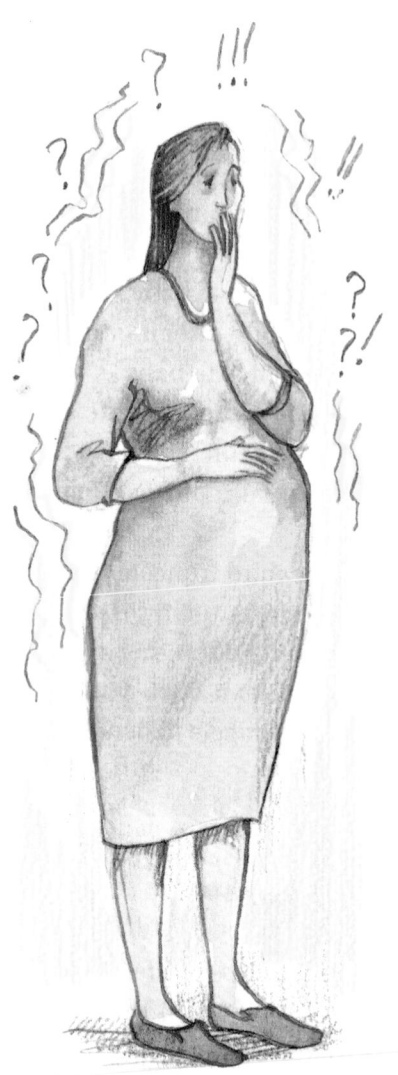

Dr. D.H. Stott's research confirms the effect of stress on the prenate. For example, he found a direct correlation between certain kinds of stresses in the mother during pregnancy and later physical and emotional problems in the child. The most problems resulted from prolonged stress in the parents' relationship. In his study of more than 1300 children and their families, Dr. Stott found that a woman in a tension-filled marriage runs a 237 percent greater risk of bearing a child with physical and emotional problems than a woman in a loving relationship. For example, a seventeen-year-old mother was coerced by her parents into marrying the father of her child and then found herself living with an alcoholic wife-batterer. She left her husband, but he tried to force her to return and even threw a brick through her window. After birth, her child vomited fresh blood and died twenty hours later. An autopsy of the infant revealed three peptic ulcers.

Prenatal stress can affect babies so profoundly as even to alter their genes. According to biologist Dr. Bruce Lipton, genes do carry hereditary information, but they can be altered (at least partially) by environmental influences. When prenates grow in a loving and peaceful environment, the "peace and love" genetic triggers are activated, thus predisposing them to physical and emotional health. In a stressful environment, the "fight or flight" triggers are pulled, actually altering the DNA and predisposing babies to physical illness and emotional problems later in life, such as aggression and violence or fear and anxiety.*

Although parents cannot eliminate all stress during pregnancy, they can minimize the harmful effects upon their baby. Psychotherapist Margaret Grant describes how she teaches her clients to do this:

> When a stressful situation occurs during a pregnancy, I teach the mother to visualize surrounding the baby with white light. I ask her to tell the baby that whatever is happening is not about the baby, that the baby is safe, and that mother will handle the situation. I find this a very successful way of teaching babies boundaries before birth.
>
> I had a client who did intense emotional release work during her pregnancy. Before each session she would visualize her baby in white light, and tell him, "This is my time and my feelings. This is not about you." Then we would proceed with her session. Four weeks after the child's birth, she came for a session with him. She repeated what she had always told him and put him down beside her. He looked at me, looked at her, closed his eyes and went to sleep. Exactly fifty-five minutes later, after sleeping through his mother's loud release of anger and fear, he opened his eyes and looked at us calmly, as if to say, "Are you finished?"

---

*"Leading edge research in cell biology reveals that 'environmental signals' are primarily responsible for selecting the genes expressed by an organism. This new perspective is in direct contrast with the established view that our fate is *controlled* by our genes. The new emphasis on nurture (environment) controlling nature (genes) focuses special attention on the importance of the maternal environment in fetal development."

However, although the environment can alter genes to the extent of creating positive or negative predispositions, so far as is currently known the environment cannot actually override genetic defects. Thus, for example, a loving and peaceful environment cannot prevent a genetic disorder such as Down's Syndrome.

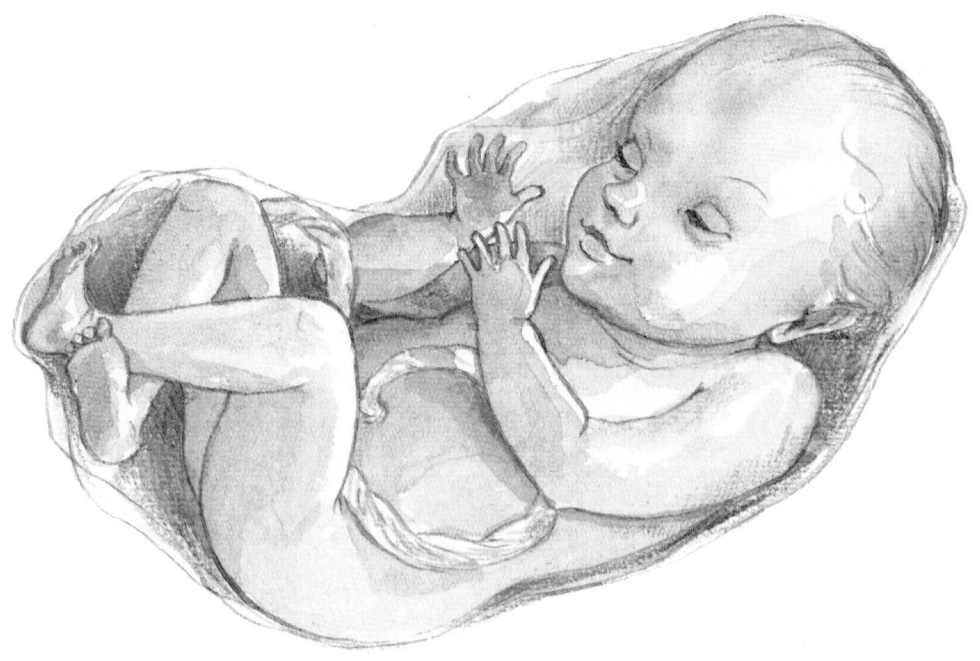

Tight Space

In addition to stresses in the parents' lives, an obvious characteristic of the third trimester is the increasing tightness of the womb. In a traumatized womb, tightness or pressure may become associated with trauma. For example, Samuel, a corporate executive, came to me (William) for therapy because he was having panic attacks. The attacks had increased every time he was promoted, and they became unbearable after he was offered the position of CEO of his company. He went to a psychiatrist who prescribed medication, but Samuel's panic attacks continued to disrupt his sleep. Samuel said,

> I feel like my office is getting smaller and smaller, and my assistants are getting larger and larger. I can't breathe very well and I'm afraid I might actually die if I get the promotion. Yet, this seems crazy because I've wanted to get to this point all my life and I'm already doing the work of a CEO. All the promotion means is a title and more money. But it feels like I have more and more pressure and less and less space.

During treatment, Samuel experienced himself going back to his third trimester. He said, "It feels like if I get any bigger I'm going to die." As it turned out, Samuel's mother had lost her first child due to stillbirth. She had not resolved this loss, and she was especially frightened after one of her doctors told her that if Samuel got any bigger he, too, might be stillborn. She really wanted Samuel but was terrified he would die in the womb. Similarly, the corporation really wanted Samuel as CEO, but he was terrified that he would die in the office. His unconscious fear of dying, imprinted upon him in his mother's womb, created the panic attacks. During treatment Samuel resolved his fear of dying. His panic attacks ceased, and he accepted the promotion to CEO. He stays in touch with me and reports that he's doing great.

The tight womb of the third trimester can affect the baby's sense of self in various ways. In a trauma-free womb, the decreasing size is experienced as safety and protection. However, in a traumatized womb, tightness may feel unsafe. Later, any situation involving psychological pressure (as in Samuel's example of a promotion) or physical pressure (such as being hugged or held tightly) may feel equally unsafe. If the baby in an unsafe womb feels constricted and trapped, the self may become identified with constriction and entrapment. As adults, such people can seem constricting and entrapping to others, even when they mean well. Or, the self may become identified with the tightness and unyieldingness of the womb, and such people may become tight and unyielding themselves.

Healing in the Third Trimester

One of the gifts of a separate sense of self is to reflect on one's experience. As the baby begins to individuate during the third trimester, any trauma that he or she has defended against emerges into awareness and is reexperienced in a more conscious and reflective way. On this basis, the baby forms a primitive sense of self and of the meaning of life. If life in the womb has been good and any trauma has been resolved, the baby experiences himself or herself as good and has a positive expectation of life. However, if life in the womb has been bad and the baby has a lot of unresolved trauma, he or she is likely to identify with the trauma. Such a baby may assume that he or she, too, is bad and may expect that life will continue to be difficult.

Because empathic presence is the greatest resource in resolving trauma, parents can help their babies immensely during the third trimester. If they recognize their baby as a conscious being who has thoughts and feelings about past experience, then the baby will not feel alone. If parents acknowledge any trauma that has occurred during the pregnancy (fights, ambivalence about the pregnancy, smoking, lack of awareness of their child as a conscious being, etc.) and ask the child's forgiveness, parent and child become partners in healing. Parents can also affirm the child's fears of birth and of life outside the womb and can pray with the child for healing.

Healing
Umbilical Trauma

We (Dennis and Sheila) were not physically present to John during his third trimester. However, it is never too late to help a child resolve prenatal trauma. For example, while he was in the womb, John suffered "umbilical trauma." This refers to the trauma that a baby suffers when toxic substances, including the mother's own stress hormones, come through the umbilical cord. In John's case, his birth father abandoned his birth mother, and she spent the months of her pregnancy homeless and under extreme stress. She smoked regularly, ate junk food, and drank alcohol.

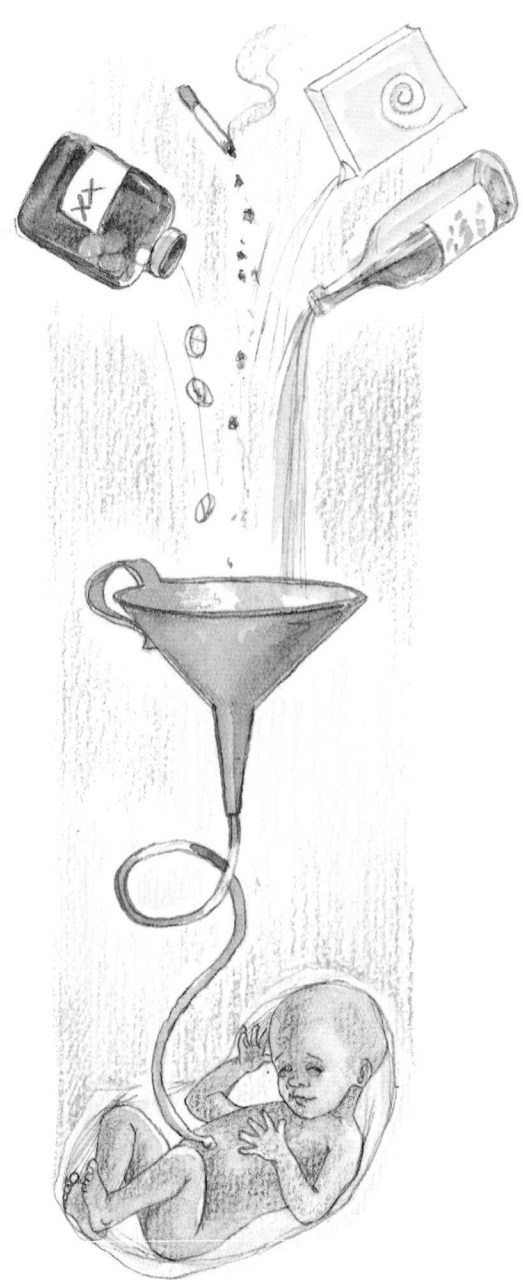

John could not protect himself from the waves of toxic chemicals (especially nicotine and alcohol) that came into him. He *tried*, as evidenced by his contracted navel, hands, and feet after birth. His body had already learned to contract and cringe in the face of intrusion or assault. Unlike most newborns, he did not spontaneously push away things he did not want. This could have become a lifelong pattern of feeling helpless to protect himself.

I (William) taught Dennis and Sheila how to help John learn healthy assertiveness. First, I encouraged John to express his feelings about his umbilical trauma, mostly through crying. We all verbalized those feelings for him. As we did so, John would stop crying and look at us in what seemed like amazement, as if to say, "How did you know?!" (During the treatment process, John's total daily crying time decreased from two or three hours per day to about ten minutes per day. I believe that a major portion of crying in babies is an effort to discharge feelings related to prenatal and perinatal trauma. Babies with no birth trauma cry an average of twenty minutes per day, and most of this crying is for the purpose of communicating their needs and discomforts.) Then, I showed Dennis and Sheila how to push gently against the bottoms of John's feet or the palms of his hands until he pushed back, cheering for him as he did so. John's hands and feet gradually opened as he developed a healthy capacity to push away what he does not want. He now has excellent boundaries.

Although John's boundaries were violated in a very obvious way, all babies need to know that they can say "Yes" and "No." Thus, when we (Dennis and Sheila) are giving retreats, we ask the group to restrain themselves from patting, poking, or pinching John. We ask that they wait to touch him until he initiates contact by reaching out in some way. Our retreatants are often quite surprised by our request, assuming that babies aren't yet capable of setting their own boundaries. Yet, from his first retreat when he was four months old, John has clearly indicated when and by whom he wants to be touched. He does this by reaching out to a person by whom he does want to be touched and by turning his head away from a person by whom he does not want to be touched.

Sometimes people ask us if and when we will tell John that he is adopted. We usually respond by saying, "John already knows. He's been telling *us* since he was three weeks old. We have thirty hours of videotaped treatment sessions during which he told us all about it." John communicates his experience of the womb and of birth in nonverbal ways, such as crying in response to specific cues, eye contact, and pushing away. Like John, we all know what it was like in the womb and at our birth, and we can receive healing as we honor that knowing.

☾ *Healing Process for Oneself*

1. You may wish to light a candle. Close your eyes and breathe deeply, breathing in God's love for you.

2. Let yourself go back to when you were in your mother's womb. Imagine yourself as a tiny being, curled up under your mother's heart.

3. Place your hands over your navel. Ask yourself when you might have experienced umbilical trauma. This might include toxic substances your mother ingested, knowingly or unknowingly. It might also include stress hormones related to events in your parents' lives, such as difficulties in their marriage, financial problems, accidents, illness, deaths of loved ones, war, or other forms of social upheaval. Perhaps your parents were simply anxious because you were their first child.

4. Use your hands to push away from your navel anything that came into you that you did not want. You might imagine Jesus, Mary, Joseph, or some other person who mediates God's healing love helping you to do this. Notice your feelings, and verbalize them if you wish. For example, as you push with your hands, you may

want to say something like, "Get out!," "Stop!" or, "This is *my* body, and I can choose what comes inside it!" If you wish, ask a friend to help you by letting you push against his or her hands.

5. Rest your hands on your navel once again, and breathe in from God what you most need. Imagine the light of God, represented by the candle, entering through your navel, and trace its journey through your entire body. Let this light replace anything negative that preceded it.

✆ *Healing Actions for Oneself*

1. For the next week, eliminate one toxic substance from your diet as a way of communicating your care to the prenate you once were that is still a part of you.

2. Lie in a warm bathtub or on a waterbed. You may wish to light a candle and play soothing music, such as Mozart, Vivaldi, or the tape series "Transitions" mentioned in Chapter 7.

3. Ask a safe person to place his or her hands lovingly on your navel and care for that part of your body.

✆ *Healing Process for Unborn Children*

This prayer can be adapted for a child who has already been born.

1. You may wish to light a candle. Breathe deeply, breathing in God's love for you and for your child.

2. One or both parents lovingly place your hands over the mother's womb. Ask your child to help you recall or become aware of any times when toxic substances may have entered his or her body through the umbilical cord. Perhaps you drank alcohol, smoked, took legal or illegal drugs, or ate unhealthy foods. Perhaps you experienced a stressful situation in which you felt overwhelmed by negative emo-

tions. Whatever comes to you, talk over the situation with your child. If it seems appropriate, ask your child's forgiveness.

3. Breathe in the healing love of God for yourself and for your child. Assure your child that you intend to do all you can to protect him or her and to care for yourself so that you will be able to transmit health to your child.

☾ *Third Trimester Game*

If your child is a baby, lay her on top of a large blanket on the floor. With two adults on each side of the blanket, slowly (take about two minutes) raise both sides of the blanket to a vertical position. Then slowly cross the sides over the baby, keeping her face uncovered to allow breathing. Stop at the slightest sign of agitation on

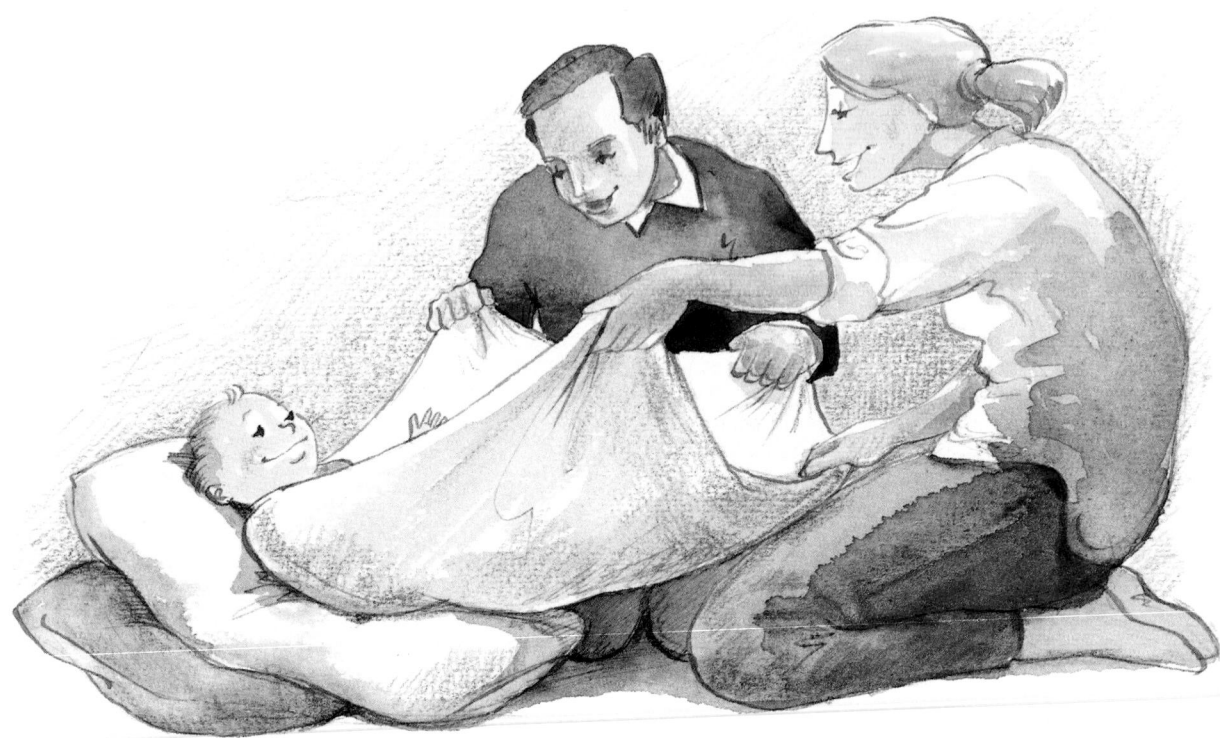

the baby's part, and pick the baby up to comfort her. Continue wrapping the blanket slowly around the baby, almost like swaddling. Gently squeeze the blanket more and more tightly around the baby's body. This will stimulate third trimester feelings, when the baby felt most tightly enclosed in the womb. This process can be very healing if it is done gently and empathically and if you stop to provide comfort whenever the baby shows any agitation.

With an older child, wrap the child as above but swing him back and forth in the blanket, sometimes tightening it. Whenever the child becomes agitated or frightened, stop the swinging and acknowledge his feelings. Afterward, invite the child to draw a picture of what he experienced.

CHAPTER 9

❦

Birth

As a newborn, John woke up screaming every night around 1:20. This was the only time each day that he woke up in this way. We learned from his birth records that he was born at 1:20 A.M. As mentioned earlier, when John was three weeks old, William treated him for birth trauma. After that first treatment session, John stopped waking up at 1:20 A.M.

When birth trauma is not treated in infancy, its effects are carried into adulthood. For example, the noted psychologist Nandor Fodor noticed that his clients had headaches, insomnia, and attacks of various fears that correlated exactly with the time and day of their birth. When they made a conscious connection between their symptoms and traumatic aspects of their birth, Dr. Fodor's clients recovered.

Birth trauma is relatively easy to identify because it is imprinted upon the body. Almost anyone can learn to look at another person and determine which physical trauma he or she experienced at birth. For example, our friend, Cris, has a left shoulder that is lower than the right. Her left eye is lower as well, and her forehead is lower on the left side. Her spine forms a *C* curve to the left. Until recently, we (Dennis, Sheila, and Matt) would not have even noticed these things, much less understood their meaning. Now we know that Cris was probably lying on her left side in the womb and experienced a difficult birth that included a lot of compression. (The side on which a baby is lying is compressed most during birth.) Her body has carried the effects of her birth into adulthood.

Similarly, I (Sheila) have indentations next to both of my eye sockets—the result of forceps that were used in my birth. The effects of birth trauma such as the use of forceps are far more than physical. For example, during a regression experience at one of William's workshops, I was lying on my back with my eyes closed. Denny placed his hands over the indentation on the left side of my head. I experienced feelings of shock and involuntarily began to back away from Denny's hand such that I

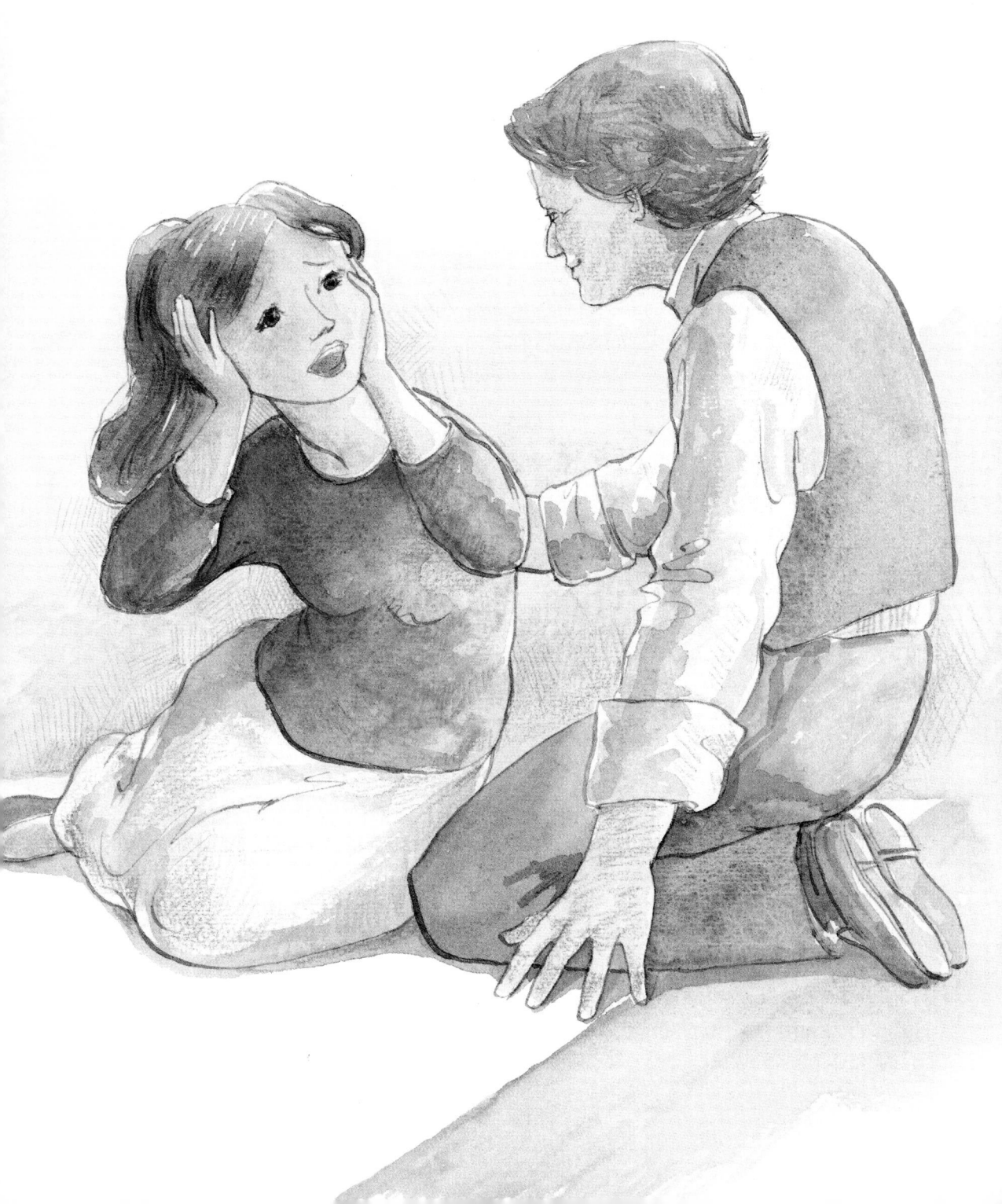

rotated about 180 degrees on the floor. I felt myself cringing with dread. I had an image of a large, cold, metal "Caterpillar" digging machine, with the arm directed at me.

William came to help Denny as he worked with me. They asked me to look into their eyes. After several minutes of loving eye contact, William asked me to push against his arm and vocalize my feelings about being intruded on by forceps. I pushed his arm away and said, "No! Get away from me. No! This is *my* space."

It is significant that the "No" I said to being intruded on by forceps during birth felt similar to the "No" I said to the intrusion that I experienced during conception, as described in Chapter 4. Although the use of forceps is almost always traumatic, it was even more so for me because it was layered upon a fear of intrusion that began at conception. Birth trauma often recapitulates prenatal trauma, and when prenatal trauma has been healed, it is easier to heal birth trauma. Perhaps because I had already resolved some of the trauma of my conception, symbolically pushing away forceps further healed my tendency to cringe and withdraw in the presence of people who are intrusive or aggressive. Later, William said it was the first time he had heard my voice without a tremor of shock from birth trauma.

The change William noted in my voice is consistent with the work of Dr. Henry Truby. By analyzing the spectrographs of the voices of newborns, he could determine which of a wide variety of prenatal and perinatal traumas they had experienced. Trauma affects our bodies, our voices, and our whole being. This is true of the trauma of birth in particular because birth is such a profoundly shocking experience, even under the best of circumstances.

Why Birth Is Shocking

We go into shock when our defenses are overwhelmed. The normal human defenses in stressful situations are fight or flight. Birth is shocking—perhaps the most shocking experience in life—because neither of these defenses will work. As contractions increase, the baby can neither flee from nor fight off the forces propelling her forward and compressing her against the pelvic opening. Does this mean that all births are traumatic?

No, despite the shocking nature of birth, about 5 percent of babies born in our culture experience little or no lasting trauma. Whether a stressful experience will cause lasting trauma depends on whether or not we are enfolded in empathic, loving presence as we go through that experience. A baby who is born to parents who are out of touch with themselves, carrying unresolved birth trauma of their own, anesthetized, intimidated by medical personnel, or otherwise emotionally unavailable to that baby is likely to sustain trauma at birth. However, a baby whose parents are aware of what their child is experiencing and who empathically communicate their awareness to the child is far less likely to sustain lasting damage, even if the birth is difficult.

For example, during my (William) son's birth, the doctors told us that Myrtle (my wife's) pelvis was too narrow and that Jamie would not be able to get out without some kind of intervention. The choices the doctors gave us were a forceps/vacuum delivery or a cesarean section. I knew either option was potentially traumatic for both Jamie and Myrtle.*

Any medical intervention can be harmful because it interferes with the cooperative effort of mother and baby to accomplish something that they are both biologically programmed to do. The first option, a forceps/vacuum delivery, would have included the use of the drug pitocin (to increase contractions), anesthesia (to decrease pain), and an episiotomy (to create more vaginal space for Jamie's head). I was concerned about this procedure because forceps can cause physical damage and a wide variety of emotional problems, ranging from Sheila's pattern of fearful withdrawal to the opposite pattern of rebellion and anti-authoritarian attitudes. As for drugs, the American Academy of Pediatrics has issued a warning that no drugs have been proven safe for unborn babies, including obstetrical drugs. The danger of obstetrical drugs is compounded by the fact that they are prescribed on the basis of the mother's weight, which means that a tiny baby receives an overdose.

When anesthesia is used during birth, it can affect neurological development, cause brain damage from hypoxia (less oxygen than is medically deemed necessary), and increase the risk of substance abuse in later life. Karr-Morse and Wiley write,

---

*One must always weigh the benefits of medical interventions against the potential for psychological traumatization. In this case, Myrtle and Jamie could have died without medical intervention. I believe that preventing loss of life or such things as brain damage or physical harm to a birthing mother are worth the psychological traumatization caused by medical interventions.

As we become more conscious of the sensitivity of the baby during and immediately following birth, the routine administration of drugs during labor and delivery, once unquestioned, is being examined in relationship to later behavioral outcomes. Several studies indicate that the use of obstetrical anesthesia during delivery may cause subtle alterations in the formation of neurons, synapses, and neural transmitters that are undetectable at birth. One seven-year study of over three thousand babies showed long-lasting effects of anesthesia on behavior and motor development. These babies were more likely to be slow to sit, stand, and walk. By age seven they lagged in language skills; their capacities for memory and judgment were also affected. Dr. Bertel Jacobson, a Swedish researcher, found a connection between adult addiction to opium and the use of opiates, barbiturates and nitrous oxide at birth.

Other studies have found that anesthesia at birth can cause such respiratory problems as emphysema, asthma, and hyperventilation. These studies confirm my experience of accompanying thousands of people during regressions. Such people will describe themselves as feeling "dazed" or "in a fog." Strange as it may sound, during many of these regressions, I and others present in the room could smell anesthesia (especially ether) being released from the person's system—anesthesia that was used thirty, forty, fifty or more years ago when the person was born.

In addition to anesthesia, other drugs can also have long-term effects. For example, when pitocin is used to induce birth or augment contractions, babies often experience a loss of control. This is because, from the baby's point of view, pitocin causes an uncontrollable increase in the frequency and intensity of contractions. This can be expressed in later life as always needing to be in control or tending to surrender control at times when it is not appropriate to do so.

Our second option, a cesarean section, was not desirable, either. A cesarean robs the baby of experiencing his own power to push his way out, which is important for self-esteem and psychological health. Thus, for example, cesarean-born babies often have trouble completing things later in life because they weren't able to complete their birth. The ideal at birth is that the baby experiences success and completion at the very first enterprise of his postuterine life. Because the primary learning style of babies is physical, what they accomplish physically translates into their inner life in terms of self-confidence.

Although cesarean delivery disrupts this process of developing self-confidence,

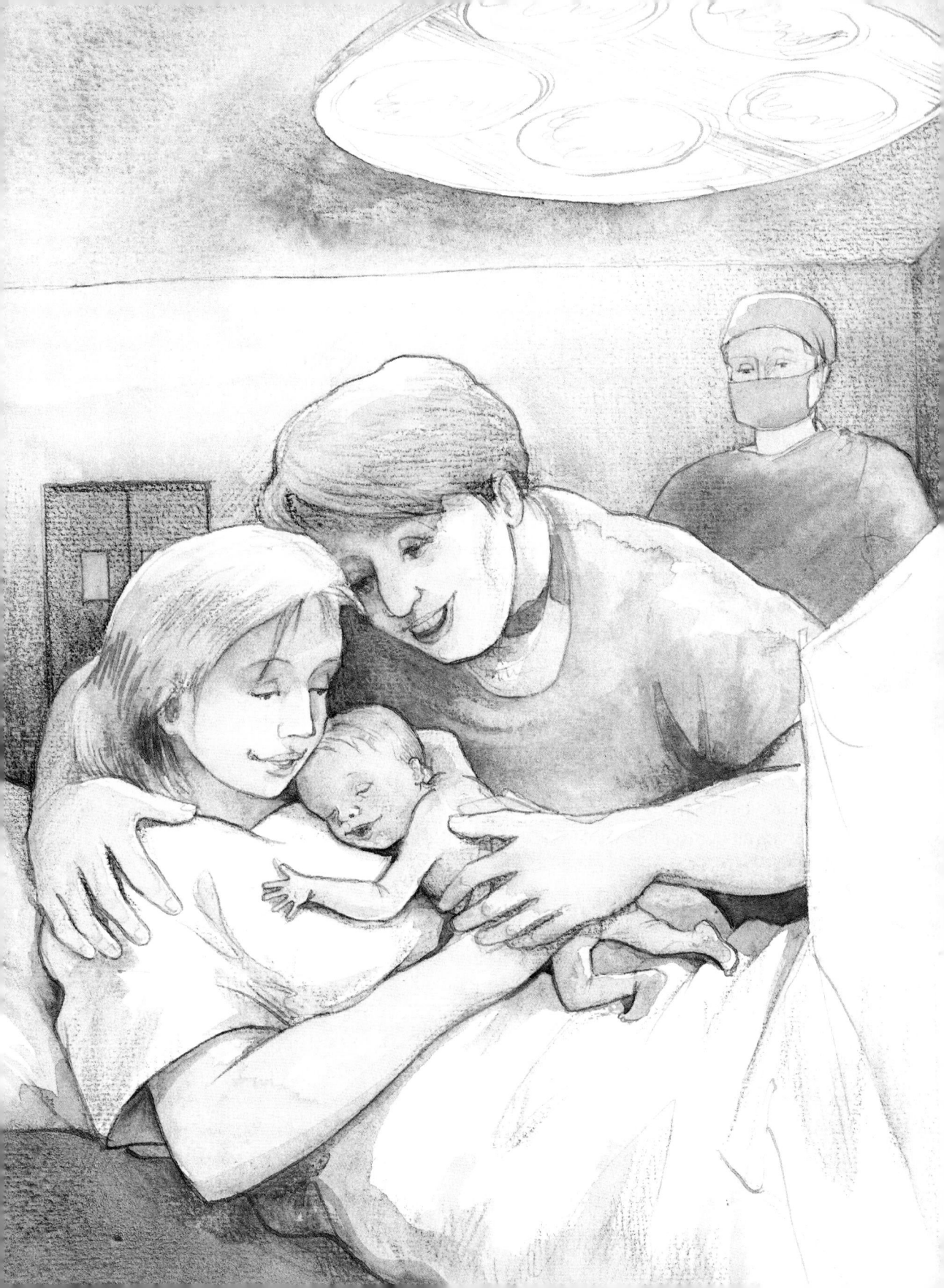

Myrtle and I decided that it was the better of our options. We did so knowing that, unfortunately, anesthesia would be used in the form of an epidural, which does enter the baby's body, although at a slower pace than general anesthesia. As we prepared ourselves, the first thing we did was to check our own well-being and preparedness. Myrtle was fine, but I felt a lot of grief about "losing" a natural birth. I cried for fifteen minutes. Then we prepared Jamie by telling him that the pelvis was too narrow for him to get through and that it was not his fault. We explained that the doctors would cut open the uterus and pick him up. Normally, we would have asked his permission and tried to intuit his answer, but in this case we didn't because it seemed that we had no other choice.

Myrtle and I remained emotionally present to Jamie throughout the surgery, empathizing with what we sensed he might be feeling and assuring him that we were with him. As soon as possible after he was out, I took him and refused all medical procedures that I knew from my own research were unnecessary. Myrtle and I kept him in our arms. We did this because we knew that one of the most traumatic experiences for newborns is to be separated from their parents for any significant amount of time.

It is separation from loving caregivers that hurts babies most, whether literal physical separation in the minutes, hours, or days after birth or lack of emotional presence at any time during the perinatal period. Such separation vastly increases the chances of impaired bonding and attachment disorders, and the likelihood of aggression and violence in later life. According to Karr-Morse and Wiley, birth complications alone do not predict violence in later life. However, if a baby experiences birth complications *and* rejection or separation from his or her mother, the potential for criminal behavior in adulthood increases greatly.

Parents Recapitulate Their Own Trauma

Most parents want to be present emotionally to their babies at birth, but sometimes their own fears and unresolved trauma get in the way. Women who are anxious about giving birth communicate stress rather than emotional presence to their babies, and this causes a higher incidence of birth complications and obstetrical interventions. In general, women tend to give birth in the way that they themselves were born, recapitulating their own trauma. For example, we videotaped a mother and later her daughter as they regressed to their births. Both were born after long hours of difficult labor involving similar complications. The videotape showed identical movements as each struggled to be born. The mother told us that *her* mother also was born after long hours of difficult labor, involving the same complications.

Moreover, other kinds of trauma are often evoked during birth. As mentioned earlier, the parents' reality permeates into the child. A common "permeation trauma" during birth is sexual abuse. As psychotherapist Dr. Michael Irving and obstetrician Dr. Bethany Hays have each observed, if the mother has been sexually abused, that memory is likely to be activated in her during delivery because giving birth can be symbolic of sexual abuse in many ways. (For example, the mother's genital area is exposed to strangers, and the movement of the child through the birth canal and resulting pain—which the mother cannot control—may be similar to the pain of sexual violation.) Not only does the mother's traumatic experience of sexual abuse permeate into the baby, but it can also interfere with the actual process of birth.

In fact, Western culture's insistence that mothers give birth lying on their backs (making labor and delivery more difficult) rather than squatting, as in most non-Western cultures, has its roots in sexual abuse. French King Louis XIV was sexually aroused by watching his mistresses give birth to his children. He forced them to lie down because he was not able to see well enough when they squatted.

What Parents Can Do

Despite all these possibilities for babies to be traumatized at birth and many more that we have not mentioned, parents can do a lot to prevent long-term negative effects. Much of what follows also applies to adoptive parents, who are also giving birth in their own way.

The first thing that all parents can do is to seek healing for themselves prior to having a child so that their own birth and other traumas will not permeate into their child. As they prepare for their child's birth, they can request a "doula," a woman caregiver whose only task is to provide emotional support for the parents during labor and delivery. Several large studies by Dr. Marshall and Phyllis Klaus and Dr. John Kennell have demonstrated the emotional and physical benefits of doulas. It seems that a woman is so emotionally open and vulnerable as she gives birth that

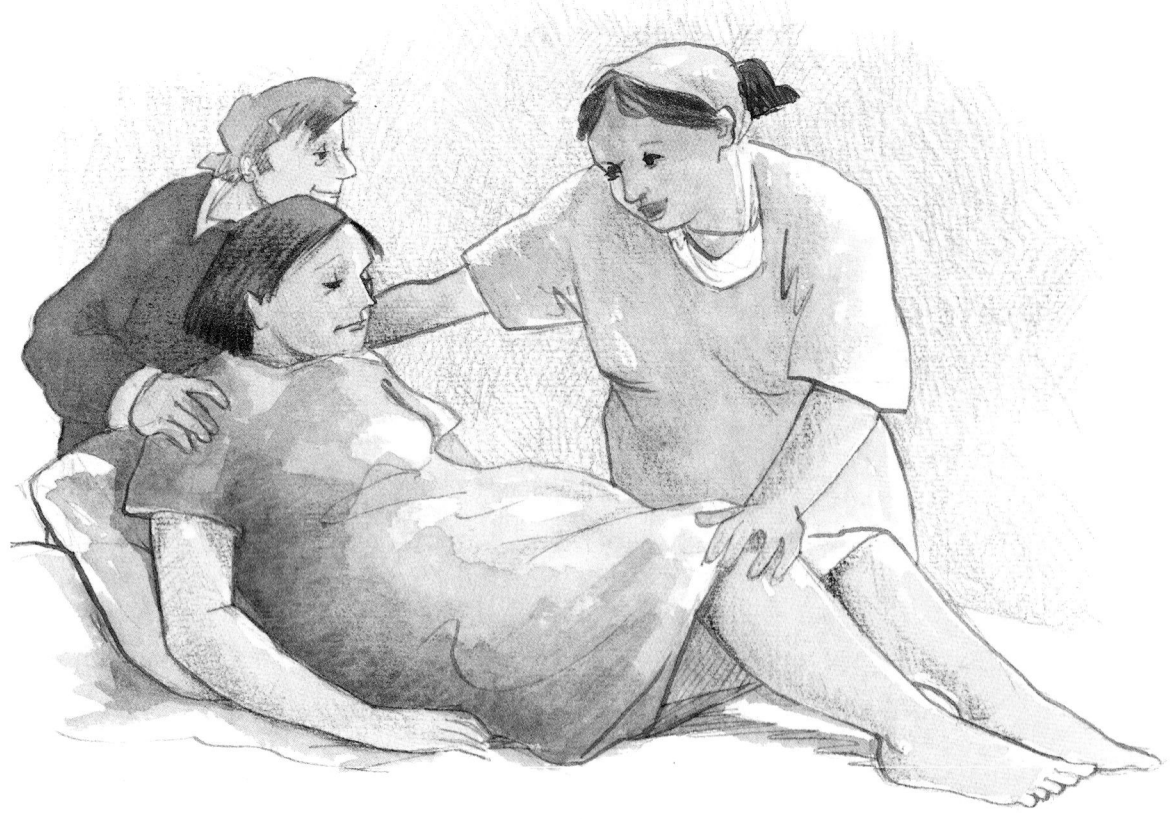

whatever happens at this time imprints deeply on her and affects future behavior. If she is unconditionally affirmed by a doula who functions as a loving mother figure, this imprints on her and can overcome years of negative messages from her own mother. It is as if she forms a new template for mothering. She will then instinctively and automatically pass on to her child the affirming love she has received, including during the birth process itself. The documented medical benefits of having a doula during birth include the reduction of first-time labor by an average of two hours, the reduction of cesarean sections by 50 percent, and the reduction of birth complications and need for pain medication.

The benefits of having a doula continue after birth. Women who have had a doula will show more maternal behaviors toward their newborns. As their children grow, these mothers are more likely to respond in unconditionally loving ways, passing on what they received from the doula. Fathers also report that having a doula helped them be more lovingly present to their wives and their new babies. Adoptive parents can replicate the benefits of having a doula. For example, we (Dennis and Sheila) deliberately surrounded ourselves with unconditionally loving mothers and fathers as we waited for a baby.

What Else Can Parents Do?

Besides seeking healing for their own hurts and enlisting the help of a doula during the birth process, other ways parents can minimize the risks of birth trauma include the following:

- They can educate themselves regarding obstetrical procedures and refuse any interventions that are not truly necessary (including circumcision, which profoundly traumatizes most boys in our culture and which a growing number of medical professionals now recognize as harmful).
- They can honestly express their feelings about any complications or medical interventions that really are necessary and take care to forgive themselves for not having a "perfect" birth.
- They can explain to their child what will happen during the birth process, and as the child is being born, they can compassionately verbalize the feelings they sense in their child.
- They can pray for healing in all the ways suggested in this book and in any others that are meaningful to them.

A child who is lovingly accompanied through birth in these ways or who is healed later of trauma brings the gift of giving birth—to the self and to others—into all later transitions in life, ultimately including death.

✆ *Healing Process for Oneself*

If we experienced trauma during birth, we can join Jesus (or God as we understand God) at Bethlehem (or another safe and welcoming birthplace) and receive love in whatever ways we most needed it during our own birth. A psychotherapist describes how she prayed with one of her clients:

Anna had felt very insecure all her life and tried to compensate by seeking upper class friends. Anna was conceived out of wedlock in a poor family. She did not want to be born because of the family's stressful circumstances. Labor was long and her birth was difficult. As I prayed for healing of her birth, Anna experienced Jesus receiving her and placing her in his mother's arms to be taken to Bethlehem. As Jesus gave her to Mary, she clearly heard him say,

> "In the eyes of the world my birth was like yours—out of wedlock, my father was not my real father and I was born in a very poor and dirty place. That is why I invite you to receive the love I received at Bethlehem."

In that moment Anna realized that the poverty of her family and the difficult circumstances of her arrival were the very things that made her birth like Jesus' birth. She felt Jesus' deep love for her right in the midst of her trauma.

For the next two weeks, Anna returned often in her imagination to Bethlehem, taking in what she needed from Mary to heal her birth. She also received another healing there, from Joseph. He gave her the love she had not received from her stepfather, who was a very angry man.

In the months that followed, Anna no longer needed to associate with wealthier people to compensate for her feelings of shame and inadequacy. She became increasingly secure and able to be herself.

Following is a prayer like the one that healed Anna:

1. You may wish to begin by reading the story of Jesus' birth in Luke 2:1–18.

2. Close your eyes and breathe deeply. If you wish, sing "Silent Night" softly to yourself, and breathe in the peace of that night. You may wish to put your hand on any part of your body where you think you may carry birth trauma.

3. Imagine yourself as a baby in the crib at the stable in Bethlehem. Scrunch up your shoulders or your hands or your toes to help you feel smaller, like a baby. Use all your senses to enter the scene. Feel the straw between your toes and the cold night air on the edge of your nostrils. Let a shiver go up and down your spine. Hear the sounds of the animals, and smell their bodies near you in the stable. See the faces of Mary and Joseph leaning over you and the starry night behind them.

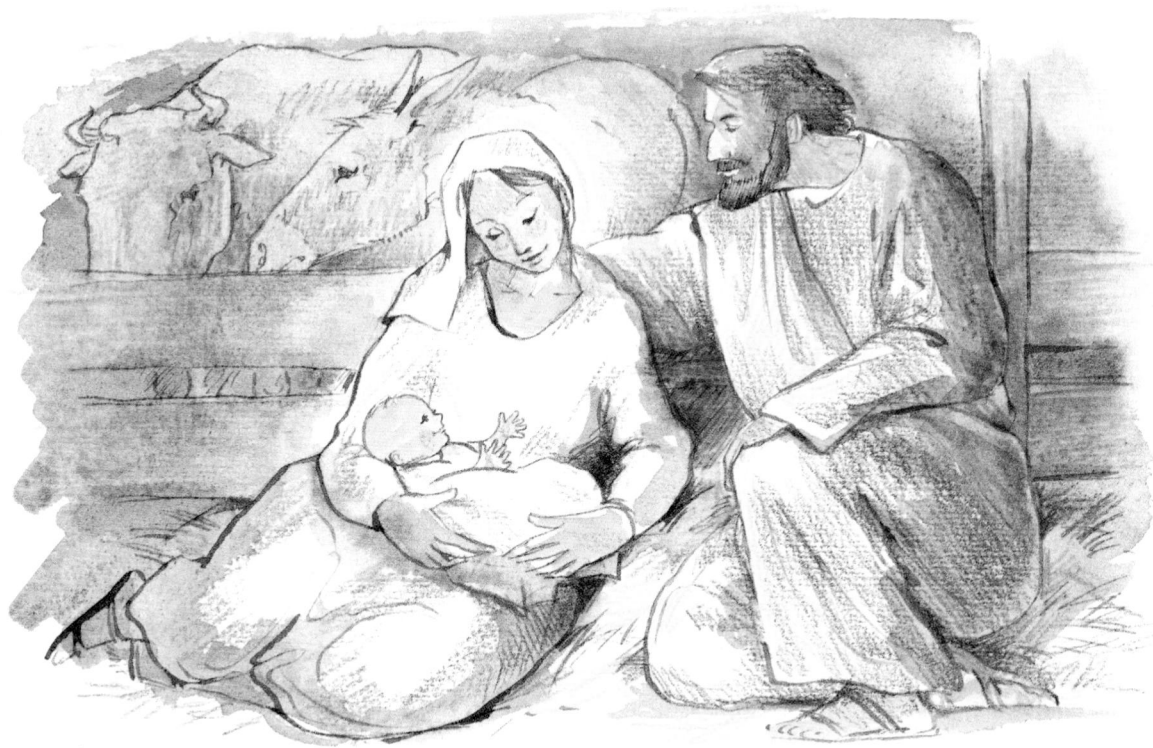

4. Become aware of whatever it is you most need. Perhaps you are cold or wet or hungry. Maybe something has frightened you. You may be exhausted from struggling to be born. Perhaps you feel alone. Whatever you are feeling, imagine that you begin to cry. You may want to let the muscles of your face contort themselves as they do when you cry.

5. Feel two hands reaching down to scoop you up and hold you. Are they the rough but loving hands of the carpenter, Joseph? Are they the smaller and gentler hands of Mary? Are they the hands of someone else?

6. For the next few minutes, let whoever holds you love you and care for you in whatever way you most need. Perhaps you need to be breast-fed, or held close and reassured, or stroked where your body was hurt in being born. Perhaps you

need to hear that you are wanted and welcome. Let the one who holds you delight in you in whatever way you most need to be delighted in.

7. You may wish to end by once more singing "Silent Night" softly to yourself, breathing in the peace of that night.

ℂ Healing Actions for Oneself

1. Ask a friend to accompany you to a playground that has a slide. Slide down, letting your friend wait for you at the bottom of the slide. Let your friend reach out and enthusiastically welcome you. Repeat this as often as you wish.

2. Find a lake or a swimming pool, get in and put your head underwater. When you long for air, come up out of the water and open your eyes. Breathe deeply, letting light and oxygen nourish you.

3. On your next birthday, plan the best possible celebration for yourself. Invite those who love you most to participate. Consciously take in their love for you.

ℂ Process for Healing a Baby's Birth

1. You may wish to begin by reading Luke 2:1–18.

2. Close your eyes and breathe deeply. If you wish, sing "Silent Night" softly to your baby as you breathe in the peace of that night.

3. In your imagination, place your baby in the crib at the stable in Bethlehem. See yourself and your baby's other parent touching and caressing your baby, with Mary and Joseph beside you.

4. Ask your baby what he or she most needs. Perhaps your baby needs protection from medication, or extra oxygen, or guidance in finding the way through the birth canal, or assurance that a cesarean delivery is not his or her fault, or to be shielded from the effects of unresolved trauma in your own life.

5. Whatever comes to you, breathe the love and protection of Jesus, Mary, and Joseph into your child.

6. You may wish to end by once more singing "Silent Night" softly to your baby, breathing in the peace of that night.

◑ *Birth Games*

1. This is a classic birth game, shared by many babies, that our John taught us (Dennis and Sheila) when he was two months old. If your child is still very small, hold her on your lap, lying on her back and with her feet against your stomach. Gently bend her legs and push her body forward toward your stomach. Encourage her to push away with her feet, saying things like, "You can push whenever *you* want to." When she pushes away, cheer for her. Be careful to hold her hands or cradle her head so that she won't fall off your lap.

2. Notice if your child seems interested in cords, such as those for telephones or appliances. If so, give him one end of a piece of cord. Hold the other end, and let him pull on it. Resist briefly, but then let him pull the cord out of your hands.

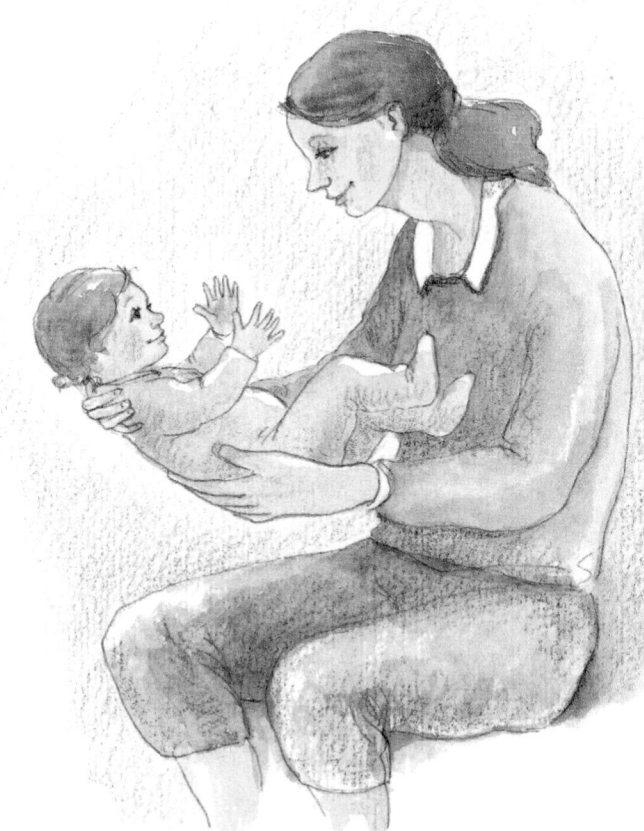

3. Use your body to form a tunnel through which your child can crawl. With a very small child, you can form the tunnel by standing or kneeling with your legs apart so the child can crawl through. Or, you can kneel, bend over, and lean on your hands so a space is formed under your

chest. Especially with an older child, you may wish to ask other family members to help form a taller, longer tunnel. Pairs of people can kneel or stand facing each other and join hands so that the child passes under their arms. As the child passes through the tunnel, cheer for the child and welcome him or her at the end.

Or, take your child to parks or other places where there are slides or tunnels to crawl through. Welcome your child at the bottom of the slide or the end of the tunnel with cheers, a big hug, and words like, "I'm so glad you're here!"

EPILOGUE

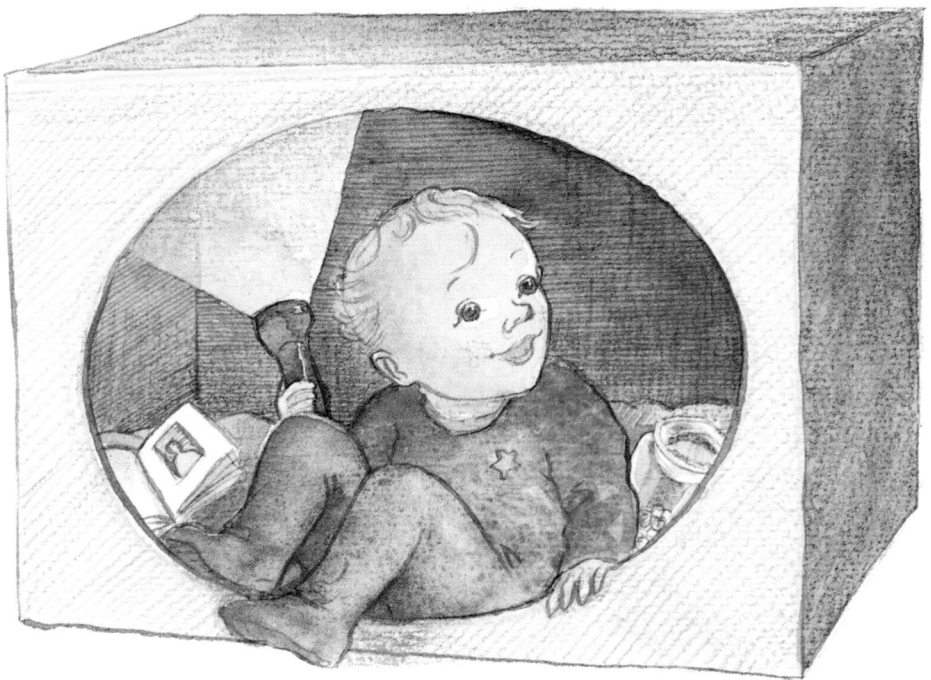

A Womb Surround

At William's suggestion, we (Dennis and Sheila) made a "womb surround" for John. A womb surround is a way of enclosing a person in such a way that he or she reexperiences being in the womb. The shawls that third world women use to carry their babies on their bodies or the American version known as a "baby sling" are a kind of womb surround. A group of people can form a womb surround by gathering around a child or an adult, or it can be made from fabric, cardboard, pillows, and the like.

After John outgrew his baby sling, we made him a womb surround from an old freezer box. We put the box on its side and cut a round hole for the entrance way. We put a soft pink quilt inside on the bottom, lined the walls with pink flannel, and draped pink silk from the ceiling. We put some of John's favorite things inside: a photo album, a jar of raisins, a flashlight, and a cassette tape player with a tape of womb sounds set to music. At least once or twice a day, John dives into his womb surround and gestures for Sheila to join him there.

It seems fitting to us that in his new womb John, who was hidden by his birth mother, now delights in pointing to the pictures in his album of ourselves, our family, and our friends welcoming him. John, who was starved by his birth mother, now giggles as he enjoys his treasured raisins in a womb that is nurturing. John can turn on his own flashlight to heal the darkness and danger he experienced in his birth mother's womb, and healthy womb sounds combined with soothing music have replaced the harsh noises of the streets and homeless shelters where his birth mother lived.

As an adopted child, John has a special need to experience himself in a safe womb with Sheila, his mother. However, all children need to experience their life after birth as being on a continuum with the safety of a healthy womb. We first understood this from Jean Liedloff's remarkable book, *The Continuum Concept*. The author spent two-and-a-half years living with a remote tribe of South American Indians. They were the happiest and most loving people she had ever met, and she attributed this to their child-rearing practices. For the first six to nine months of life, their children are in constant contact with the body of their mother or another caring adult. They sleep with their parents and are breast-fed as often as they wish.

Thus, these children's lives after birth maintain the intimate closeness with their mother that they experienced in the womb. They are never put in cribs, baby holders, playpens, or other containers. Rather, the mother watches for signals of the child's gradually emerging desire for independence, and only then does she put him down to crawl or walk on his own.*

Because these children's early lives maintain continuity with the safety and intimacy of the womb, they are likely to carry within themselves an inner womb

---

*Liedloff's ideas are gaining acceptance in North America, and have contributed to a model of parenting known as "attachment parenting." On pages 137–138, we have listed resources for those who want to explore attachment parenting.

surround to which they can always return. Like John, we all need a womb surround that is ready and waiting for us. I (Matt) create one for myself each evening before I fall asleep. I get into a fetal position and imagine myself in a safe womb filled with the presence of the Holy Spirit. I breathe in the womb's warmth and protection and breathe out any tension from the day. I can return to this womb surround any time I need to feel safe and protected. Perhaps I will even go there as I prepare to die. Dr. Rachel Naomi Remen tells the following story of one of her cancer patients:

> The second man, caught up in rage at cancer and its treatment, responded to the question "What do you think may be needed for your healing?" with a terse "Nothing!" Taking his statement at face value, I asked him to describe "nothing" to me. "Unending darkness," he said. . . . I encouraged him to close his eyes and experience it.
>
> As his face became more and more relaxed, I asked him how he was feeling. . . .
>
> The darkness is all around me. . . .
> I'm not falling. It holds me. I am held in darkness.
> Wrapped in darkness.
> The darkness is . . . soft . . . almost tender.
> It's safe here.
> I needed to feel safe. I haven't relaxed since I got the diagnosis. I can rest. I am so tired.
> No pain here. No hunger. No need.
>
> After a while, he commented that he could hear a sound "like a great heartbeat." It was deeply comforting.
>
> I encouraged him to lean up against it. To rest. Soon he began to weep softly, saying, "Mama, mama."

As light represents the archetype of masculine energy, darkness suggests the power of the feminine, and it makes an intuitive sense that the *experience* of healing may be associated with darkness. Darkness is a condition of the beginning. The body first comes into being in darkness. It is nurtured, as a seed, in darkness. Some people may find their healing in remembering the beginning.

❧❧

Chart of Fetal Development

Growth and Changes During Pregnancy

0–14 Weeks (First Trimester)

Woman

- Your period stops or is light.
- You may have nausea and vomiting. These usually go away by the end of this time.
- Your breasts become larger. They may be tender.
- Your nipples may stick out more.
- You may have to urinate more often.

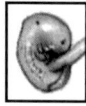

Week 4 (actual size)

Fetus

- The heart begins to beat.
- Bones appear; the head, arms, fingers, legs, and toes form.
- The major organs and nervous system form.
- The placenta forms.
- Hair starts to grow.
- 20 buds for future teeth appear.
- By the end of this time, the fetus is about 4 inches long and weighs just over 1 ounce.

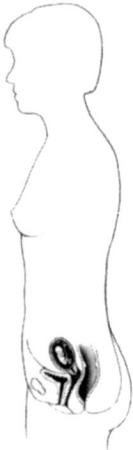

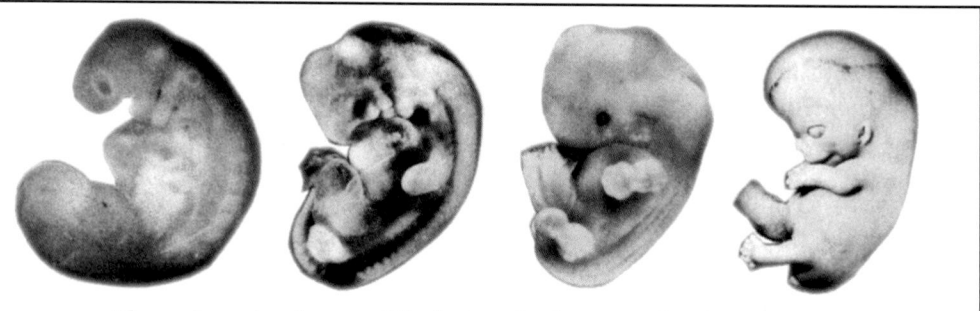

The embryo develops rapidly during the first 8 weeks of pregnancy.

PHOTOS COURTESY OF CARNEGIE INSTITUTION OF WASHINGTON.

14–28 Weeks (Second Trimester)

Woman

- Your abdomen begins to swell. Your uterus will be near your ribs by the end of this time.
- The skin on your abdomen and breasts stretches. You may see stretch marks.
- At about 16–20 weeks, you may start to feel the fetus move.
- You may get a dark line from the navel down the middle of the abdomen, or you may get brown, uneven marks on your face. Your areolas, the brown area around your nipples, may darken.

Fetus

- The fetus grows quickly from now until birth.
- The organs develop further.
- Eyebrows and fingernails form.
- The skin is wrinkled and covered with fine hair.
- The fetus moves, kicks, sleeps, and wakes. It can swallow, hear, and pass urine.
- By the end of this time, the fetus is about 11–14 inches long and weighs about 2–2½ pounds.

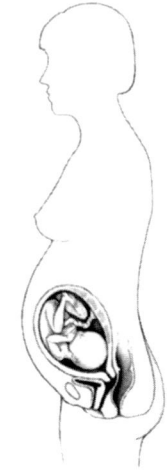

28–40 Weeks (Third Trimester)

Woman

- You can feel the movements of the fetus more strongly.
- You may have abdominal pains. These may be false or true labor pains.
- You may feel short of breath as the uterus pushes against the diaphragm, a flat, strong muscle that aids in breathing. Toward the end of this time the baby's position may drop lower in your abdomen, which will make it easier for you to breathe.
- When the baby drops, you may need to urinate more often.
- Yellow, watery fluid called colostrum may leak from your nipples.
- Your navel may stick out.
- Your cervix may begin to thin out and open slightly.

Fetus

- The fetus kicks and stretches, but as it gets bigger it has less room to move.
- Fine body hair disappears.
- Bones harden, but bones of the head are soft and flexible for delivery.
- The fetus usually settles into a good position for birth.
- At 40 weeks, the fetus will be full term. It is about 20 inches long and weighs 6–9 pounds.

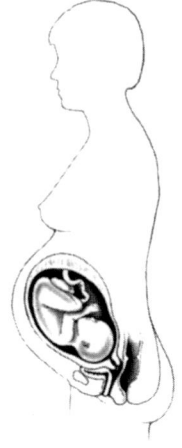

The Growth and Development of the Fetus

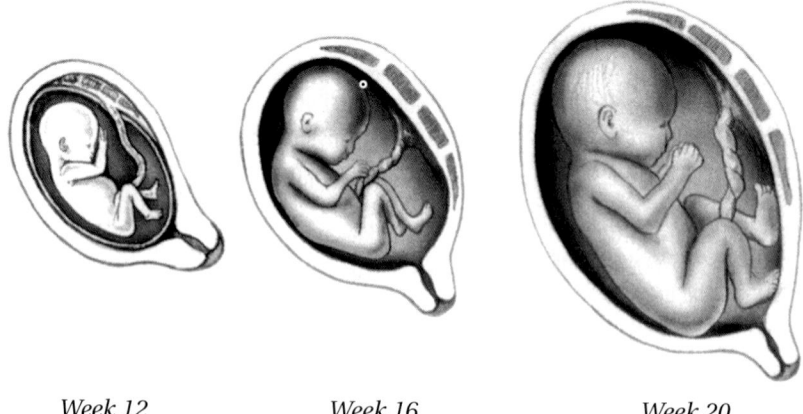

Week 12   *Week 16*   *Week 20*

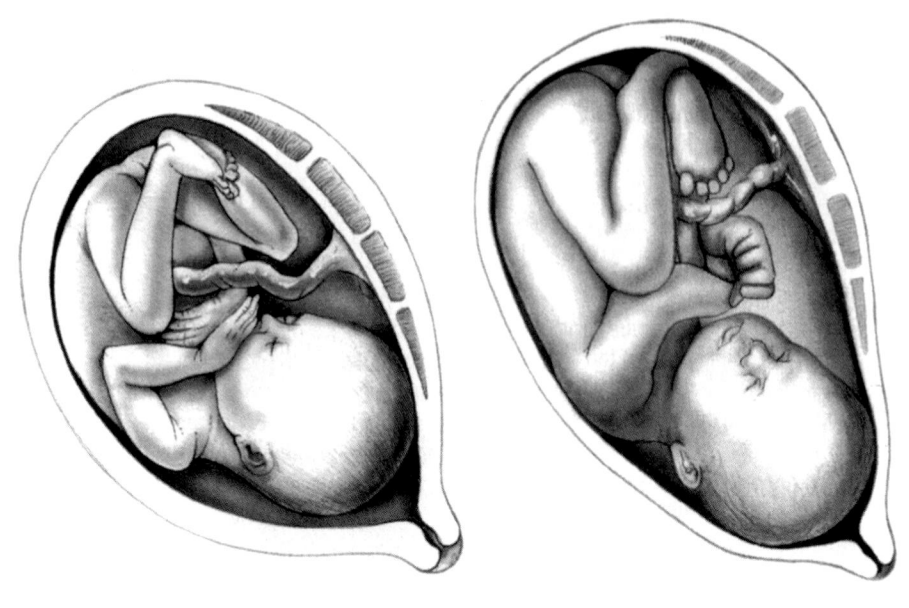

Week 32   *Week 36*

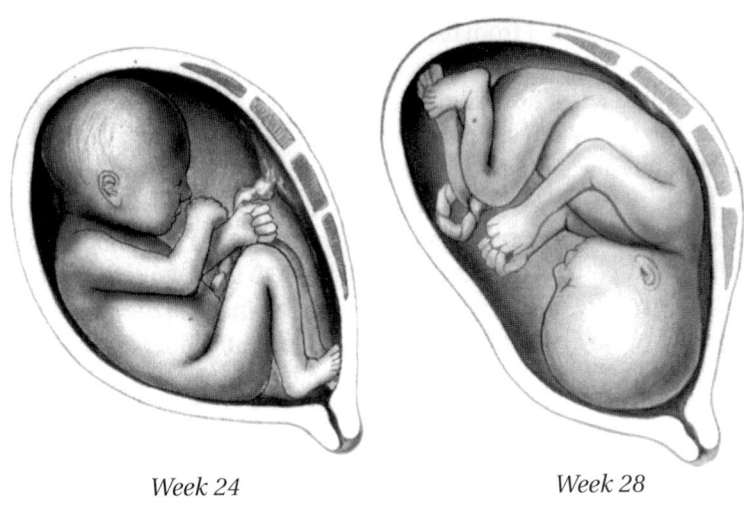

Week 24   *Week 28*

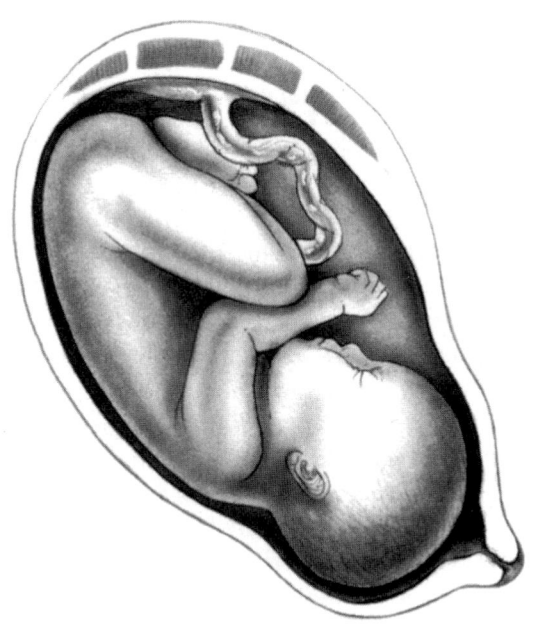

Week 40

Process for Group Sharing

Following is a suggested format for using this book as a course with a wide variety of groups, including expectant parents. The course can have eight sessions (one for each chapter, beginning with Chapter 2), or it can be shortened to suit the needs of the group. Each member of the group will need a copy of this book.

This format takes one-and-a-half to two hours for each session. Feel free to vary the format as needed. Normally, groups meet once per week, but you may wish to vary the frequency of meetings. For example, you may wish to meet every two weeks, or you may wish to have several sessions over one weekend.

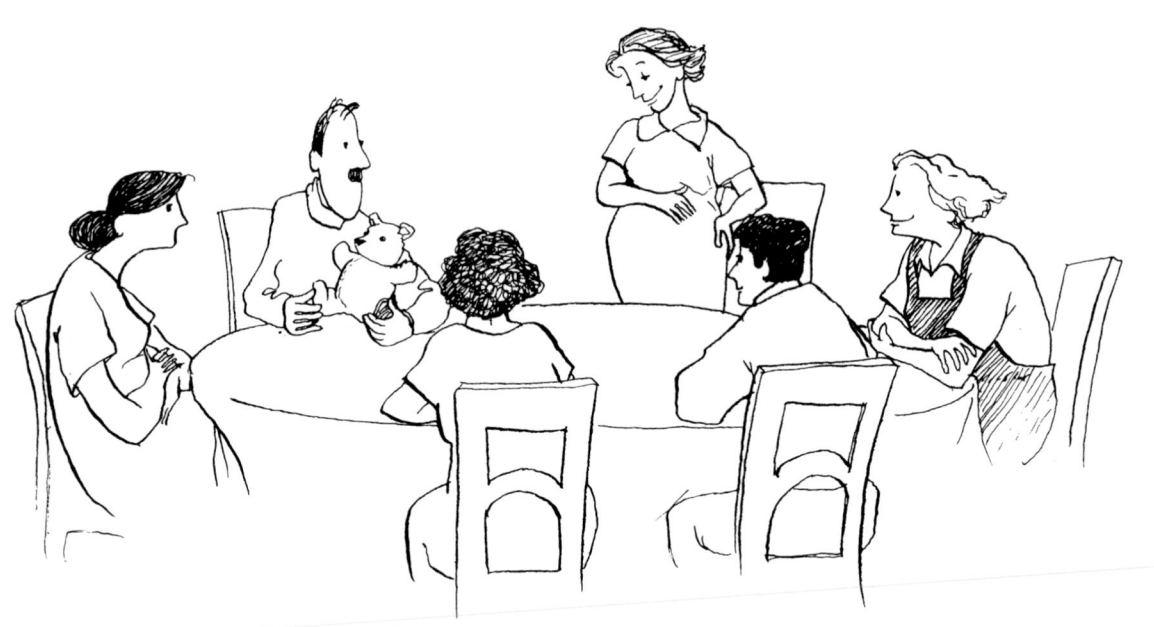

I. Group Meetings

   A. Common Opening Prayer (5 minutes)

   B. Review of This Week's Chapter (20–30 minutes)
      Beginning with Chapter 2, review this week's chapter in the book, and do the Healing Process for Oneself at the end of the chapter. (Prior to the first session, participants may wish to read Chapter 1.)

   C. Silent Reflection (3 minutes)
      Quiet time to get in touch with what part of this week's chapter moved your heart most deeply.

   D. Guided Journaling (Optional—10 minutes)
      1. Write down what is in your heart. Write to Jesus or to God as you understand God in the way that you would write a letter to your best friend, sharing what you feel most deeply. Don't worry about having the "right" words, but only try to share your heart. If you find it more helpful, draw a picture rather than write a letter.
      2. Now get in touch with how God is responding to you, as God speaks to you from within. You might do this by asking what is the most loving response that Jesus or God as you understand God could possibly make to you in response to what you have just shared.
      3. Write what you think might be God's response. Perhaps it will be just one word or one sentence, or perhaps it will be a simple drawing. You can be sure that anything you write or draw that helps you to know more that you are loved is at least part of what God wants to say to you.

   E. Companion Sharing (5 minutes minimum for each person to share his or her reaction to this week's chapter and to the home experiences during the past week.) By the second session, each person should choose one or two companions for companion sharing and companion prayer. If possible, companions should remain together throughout the course.
      1. Share with your companion as much as you wish of what is in your heart from this week's presentation. Perhaps you will want to share what you have just written or drawn during the guided journaling.

2. Share with your companion your experience at home since you last met, especially your prayer and journaling.

3. Share with your companion what you are most grateful for now and how you need help from God.

F. Companion Prayer (5–10 minutes of prayer for each person)
Pray for your companion as Jesus or God as you understand God would pray. Give thanks for whatever your companion is most grateful for, and pray for whatever healing your companion most wants. Then reverse roles, and let your companion pray for you.

G. Group Sharing and Games (Optional—15 minutes minimum)
Share with the whole group your response to this week's presentation and your experience at home since you last met. Some people may wish to share from their journals. You may wish to return to any of the games suggested for children at the end of each chapter and do them with one another as a group.

H. Closing Snack and Celebration
An open-ended time to enjoy one another and to continue sharing.

II. Preparation at Home Between Group Meetings

A. Daily Healing Prayer (10 minutes or as long as you wish)
Each day, do the Healing Process at the end of that week's chapter. For example, each day of the first week do the process at the end of Chapter 2; each day of the second week do the process at the end of Chapter 3; and so on.

B. Daily Journal (10 minutes)
1. In writing or through a drawing, share with Jesus or with God as you understand God when during this prayer or during the day your heart was deeply moved.
2. Write or draw in your journal how Jesus or God responds to what you have shared. One way to get in touch with God's response is to write or draw the most loving response you can imagine.

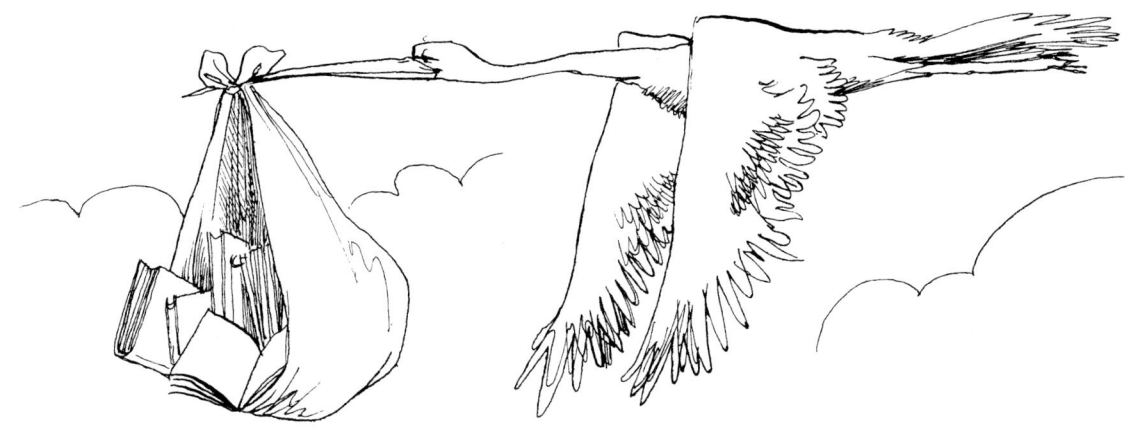

Recommended Resources

APPPAH (Association for Pre- and Perinatal Psychology and Health), 340 Colony Rd., P.O. Box 994, Geyserville, CA 95441, tel. (707)857-4041, fax (707)857-4042, www.birthpsychology.com. APPPAH publishes a catalogue of 100 books and video-tapes on the psychology of prenates and newborns, pregnancy, childbirth, infancy, parenting, and trauma resolution.

Heidi Britz-Crecelius, *Children at Play* (Rochester, VT: Park Street Press, 1996). Exquisite book, in the tradition of Waldorf education, on supporting the inner meaning and integrity of children's play.

Peter Campbell and Edwin McMahon, *Teaching Children to Focus* (interview with Marianne Thompson) and *How Adults Can Listen to Children in a Focusing Way* (interview with Gloria Brunix). Short booklets on how parents and others can help children learn to be with their feelings as they are carried in the body. Available from Institute for Bio-Spiritual Research, P.O. Box 741137, Arvada, CO 80006-1137, (303) 427-5311.

Jean Liedloff, *The Continuum Concept* (New York: Addison Wesley, 1977). Classic book on a newborn's need for a continuum with life in the womb, in the form of constant or nearly constant bodily contact with care givers.

William and Martha Sears, *The Baby Book: Everything You Need to Know About Your Baby—From Birth to Age Two* (New York: Little, Brown & Co., 1993). Guide for parents that emphasizes attachment parenting, by a widely respected mainstream pediatrician and nurse. This book is written with wisdom, love, and humor, and avoids "shoulding" parents. Includes a chapter on "Babywearing: The Art and Science of Carrying Your Baby."

Penny Simkin, *Pregnancy, Childbirth, and the Newborn* (New York: Simon & Schuster, 1991). Highly recommended source of information on the prenatal and perinatal period.

The Wellspring Review and Catalogue. Quarterly in-depth review of books for parents and children, based on attachment parenting and a holistic lifestyle. Wellness Associates, 123 Wildwood Trail, Afton, VA 22920, (800)484-3171, code 8998.

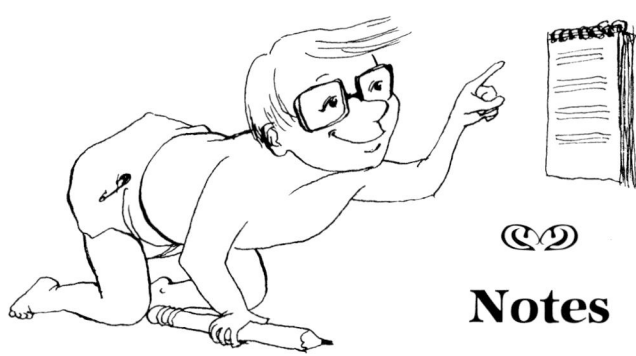

Notes

Chapter 1

Page 1: Quote is from Robin Karr-Morse and Meredith S. Wiley, *Ghosts from the Nursery: Tracing the Roots of Violence* (New York: Atlantic Monthly Press, 1997), p. 53.

Page 2: R.D. Laing, *The Facts of Life* (New York: Penguin, 1977), p. 36. One reason early trauma creates a template is that trauma alters the developing brain. Certain types of stimulation, such as anger and violence, sensitize certain brain cells, and the brain then organizes itself around those types of stimulation. Cf. Karr-Morse and Wiley, op. cit., pp. 158–170.

Pages 5–7: Here and elsewhere, we report memories of prenatal and perinatal experiences. We acknowledge the current controversy over the validity of "recovered memories" (previously repressed memories of traumatic events in early life). Some claims of recovered memories may not be historically accurate. We believe that in the majority of cases such memories are basically accurate, and in many cases they can be verified. Two such examples are William's story reported here of birth memories verified by hospital records, and Graham Farrant's story verified by his mother and by research at the Karolinska Institute (see pp. 53, 64). Regarding verification research, see David Chamberlain, *Babies Remember Birth* (Los Angeles: Jeremy P. Tarcher, 1988), Chapter 8 and William Emerson, "The Physical and Psychological Impacts of Obstetrical Interventions," (Petaluma: Emerson Training Seminars, 1996), pp. 5–12.

Whether a memory is historically accurate or whether it is symbolic, it represents a real need for healing in the person's life. Healing happens when the person receives healing into whatever they recall.

Page 11: Experiment involving shared feelings between mother and child cited in Thomas Verny, *The Secret Life of the Unborn Child* (New York: Summit, 1981), p. 76.

Page 13: *An Ounce of Prevention: Toward an Understanding of the Causes of Violence* (State of California Commission on Crime Control and Violence Prevention, 1981).

For research on circumcision, contact Doctors Opposing Circumcision (DOC), 2442 NW Market St., S–42, Seattle, WA 98107 and NOCIRC, P.O. Box 2512, San Anselmo, CA 94979.

On listening to babies when they cry, see Aletha Solter, *Tears and Tantrums* (Goleta, CA: Shining Starr Press), 1998.

Research connecting lack of attachment in early life to violence in later life is cited in Karr-Morse and Wiley, op. cit. See also Ken Magid and Carole McKelvey, *High Risk: Children Without a Conscience* (New York: Bantam, 1987).

Page 14: Results of the Hello Baby program reported in Beatriz Manrique et. al., "A Controlled Experiment in Prenatal Enrichment with 684 Families in Caracas, Venezuela: Results to Age Six," *Journal of Prenatal and Perinatal Psychology and Health*, 12:3–4 (Spring, 1998), pp. 209–234.

Page 15: For children's memory of prenatal and perinatal experience, see David Chamberlain, *The Mind of Your Newborn Baby* (Berkeley: North Atlantic Books, 1998), Chapter 7; and Sarah Hinze, *Coming from the Light* (New York: Pocket Books, 1994).

Page 16: Raymond Moody's map of near-death experiences reported in *Life After Life* (New York: Bantam, 1975).

Quote is from David Chamberlain, "Prenatal Receptivity and Intelligence," *Journal of Prenatal and Perinatal Psychology and Health*, 12:3–4 (Spring, 1998), p. 100.

Page 17: Larry Dossey, *Healing Words: The Power of Prayer and the Practice of Medicine* (San Francisco: Harper, 1993). Quote is from a letter to Dr. Martin Parmentier, December 3, 1994. Used with Dr. Dossey's permission.

Chapter 2

Page 20: Robert Coles, "Touching and Being Touched," *The Dial* (December, 1980), pp. 26–27.

Page 23: L.R. Propst, "The Comparative Efficacy of Religious and Nonreligious Imagery for the Treatment of Mild Depression in Religious Individuals," *Cognitive Therapy and Research*, 4:2 (1980), pp. 167–178.

Page 24: Louis J. Puhl (Ed.), *The Spiritual Exercises of St. Ignatius* (Chicago: Loyola University Press), 1951.

Page 27: Quote from Ignatius is from Puhl, op. cit., #112.

Page 28: Raymond Brown, *The Birth of the Messiah* (New York: Doubleday, 1977), p. 515. See also pp. 188–89, 216–17, 226–27. In *A Marginal Jew: Rethinking the Historical Jesus* (New York: Doubleday, 1991), Vol. I, John P. Meier writes,

While Jesus' birth in Bethlehem cannot be positively ruled out (one can rarely "prove a negative" in ancient history), we must accept the fact that the predominant view in the Gospels and Acts is that Jesus came from Nazareth and—apart from Chapters 1–2 of Matthew and Luke—only from Nazareth. The somewhat contorted or suspect ways in which Matthew and Luke reconcile the dominant Nazareth tradition with the special Bethlehem tradition of their Infancy Narratives may indicate that Jesus' birth at Bethlehem is to be taken not as a historical fact but as a *theologoumenon*, i.e., as a theological affirmation (e.g., Jesus is the true Son of David, the prophesied Royal Messiah) put into the form of an apparently historical narrative. One must admit, though, that on this point certitude is not to be had. (p. 216; see also 214–215)

Marcus Borg writes, ". . . Jesus was probably born in Nazareth, not Bethlehem." In Borg, *Meeting Jesus Again for the First Time* (San Francisco: Harper, 1994), pp. 23–24.

Page 29: Antonio Madrid and M. Xavier McPhee, "The Treatment of Pediatric Asthma through Maternal/Infant Bonding in Hypnosis," *The PPPANA Journal* (Spring, 1985), pp. 4–6. Although Dr. Madrid used hypnosis in the cases cited, in personal conversation with one of the authors on September 15, 1998, he expressed his opinion that hypnosis is not necessary and that healing prayer or other methods of using imagery could accomplish the same result because they access the same part of a person's consciousness as does hypnosis.

Chapter 3

Page 33: Joan Fitzherbert, "The Source of Man's 'Intimations of Immortality,'" *British Journal of Psychiatry*, 110 (1964), pp. 859–862.

Page 38: In Christian theology, baptism is regarded as the usual means for effecting the kind of complete transformation described here as the ideal resolution of divine homesickness, in which the indwelling of God permeates every aspect of a person's life. However, the Roman Catholic church recognizes that God can give this same grace to any human being, Christian or not. "Since Christ died for all, and since all men are called to one and the same destiny, which is divine, we must hold that the Holy Spirit offers to all the possibility of being made partakers, in a way known to God, of the Paschal mystery." Austin P. Flannery, O.P. (Ed.), *The Documents of Vatican II*, (New York: Pillar Books, 1975), "Gaudium et Spes," 22:5; quoted in the English translation of the *Catechism of the Catholic Church* (Washington, DC: United States Catholic Conference, Inc.—Libreria Editrice Vaticana, 1994), in the section on baptism of desire, #1260.

Chapter 4

Page 48: Dossey, *Healing Words*, op. cit., p. 49; for role of love and compassion in nonlocal communication, see pp. 51–53.

For examples of babies' ability to communicate across space and time, see Hinze, op. cit.

Page 49: Candace Pert, *Molecules of Emotion* (New York: Scribner), 1997; David Chamberlain, "The Outer Limits of Memory," *Noetic Sciences Review* (Autumn, 1990), pp. 4–13; Rupert Sheldrake, *The Presence of the Past* (New York: Times Books/Random House, l988) and his interview with Michael Toms, "The Past Is Present" (San Francisco: New Dimensions, l994).

Page 53: Steven Raymond, "Cellular Consciousness and Conception: An Interview with Dr. Graham Farrant," *Pre- & Perinatal Psychology News*, II:2 (Summer, 1988), reprinted in *The Journal of Christian Healing*, 11:3 (Fall, 1989), pp. 17–23.

Page 57: T.J. Cicero, "Effects of Paternal Alcohol on Offspring Development," *Alcohol Health and Research World, National Institute on Alcohol Use and Alcoholism*, 18:1 (January 1994), pp. 37–41; and N. Day and G. Richardson, "Comparative Teratogenicity of Alcohol and Other Drugs," *Alcohol Health and Research World, National Institute on Alcohol Use and Alcoholism*, 18:1 (January 1994), pp. 42–48.

Chapter 5

Page 64: For the impact of trauma on developing physical systems, see William Emerson, *Pre- and Perinatal Stages* (Petaluma, CA: Emerson Training Seminars, 1998, unpublished manuscript); Keith L. Moore, *The Developing Human*, 4th Edition (Philadelphia: W.B. Saunders, 1988).

Pages 68–69: For the effects of nicotine, alcohol and other drugs on the prenate, see Karr-Morse and Wiley, op. cit., Chapter 3. Quote is from pp. 60 and 62.

Page 69: Andrew Feldmar, "The Embryology of Consciousness: What Is a Normal Pregnancy?" in David Mall and Walter Watts (Eds.), *The Psychological Aspects of Abortion* (Washington, DC: Univ. Publications of America, 1979), pp. 15–24.

Chapter 6

Pages 77–78: Incidence of miscarriage and abortion from U.S. Bureau of the Census, Statistical Abstract of the U.S., 1997, (117th Edition), Washington, DC, 1997. Incidence of stillbirth from Larry G. Peppers and Ronald J. Knapp, *Motherhood and Mourning* (New York: Praeger, 1980), p. 14. As of 1997, the National Institutes of Health Neonatal Statistics reports the incidence of stillbirth as 3 per 1,000 live births. Incidence of twins from Louis G. Keith, *Multiple Pregnancy, Epidemiology, Gestation and Perinatal Outcome* (Pearl River, NY: Parthenon Publishing Group, 1995), and Elizabeth Noble, *Having Twins* (Boston: Houghton Mifflin, 1991).

Chapter 7

Page 87: Daniel J. O'Hanlon, S.J., "Integration of Christian Practices: A Western Christian Looks East," *Studies in the Spirituality of Jesuits* (May 1984), 10–11.

Pages 89–90: Quote is from Chamberlain, op. cit., p. 55.

Page 91: Dr. Veldman's work reported in S.N. Bauer, "Science of Touch and Feeling Has Great Import for Preborn," *St. Cloud Visitor*, 71:24 (November 11, 1982), pp. 1 and 11.

    Henry M. Truby and John Lind, "Cry Sounds of the Newborn Infant," in John Lind (Ed.), "The Newborn Infant Cry," *Acta Paediatrica Scandinavica* (Supplement), 163 (1965).

Pages 91–92: Babies' response to music reported by Michele Clements, "Observations on Certain Aspects of Neonatal Behavior in Response to Auditory Stimuli," paper presented at the Fifth International Congress of Psychosomatic Obstetrics and Gynecology, Rome, 1977.

Chapter 8

Page 99: Chamberlain, op. cit., p. 210; Beatriz Manrique, "Breaking the Cycle of Violence," presented at the 1995 International Congress of the Association for Pre- and Perinatal Psychology and Health.

Pages 99–100: Exercises for prenates described in F. Rene Van de Carr and Marc Lehrer, *While You Are Expecting: Your Own Prenatal Classroom* (Atlanta: Humanics Trade, 1997). Story of sixteen-month-old is from F. Rene Van de Carr and Marc Lehrer, "Prenatal University: Commitment to Fetal-Family Bonding and the Strengthening of the Family Unit as an Educational Institution," *Journal of Prenatal and Perinatal Psychology and Health*, 12:3–4 (Spring 1998), pp. 119–134.

Page 100: Anthony DeCasper and Melanie Spence, "Prenatal Maternal Speech Influences Newborn's Perception of Speech Sounds," *Infant Behavior and Development*, 9, 1986, pp. 133–150.

Pages 100–101: William R. Emerson, "Trauma and Spirituality," (Petaluma, CA: Emerson Training Seminars, 1997).

Pages 102–103: D.H. Stott, "Follow-up Study from Birth of the Effects of Pre-Natal Stresses," *Devel. Med. Child Neurol.*, 15 (1973), pp. 770–787. See also Verny, op. cit., pp. 87–88, and Charles Spezzano, "Prenatal Psychology: Pregnant with Questions," *Psychology Today*, (May 1981), pp. 49–57.

Page 103: Bruce H. Lipton, "Nature, Nurture and the Power of Love," *Journal of Prenatal and Perinatal Psychology and Health*, 13:1 (Fall 1998), pp. 3–10; quote is from the abstract on p. 3. See also Karr-Morse and Wiley, op.cit., pp. 10 and 79–80.

For the relationship of prenatal stress and violence, see Karr-Morse and Wiley, op. cit., pp. 93–95.

Page 107: Average crying time in babies reported in William Emerson, "The Physical and Psychological Impacts of Obstetrical Interventions," (Petaluma: Emerson Training Seminars, 1996), p. 16.

Chapter 9

Page 112: Nandor Fodor, *The Search for the Beloved* (New Hyde Park: University Books, 1949).

Page 114: Personal conversation between Henry Truby and David Chamberlain, reported in Chamberlain, op. cit., pp. 68–69.

Page 116: Quote regarding anesthesia from Karr-Morse and Wiley, op. cit., p. 76.

Relationship between anesthesia and respiratory problems reported in David Cheek, "Maladjustment Patterns Apparently Related to Imprinting at Birth," *Amer. J. of Clinical Hypnosis*, 18:2 (1975), pp. 75–82.

Page 118: Relationship of criminal behavior to a combination of birth complications and maternal separation or rejection reported in Karr-Morse and Wiley, op. cit., pp. 90–91.

Page 119: Michael Irving, "Sexual Assault and Birth Trauma: Interrelated Issues," *Pre- and Perinatal Psychology Journal*, 11:4 (Summer 1997), pp. 215–250; Dr. Bethany Hays, video-taped interview with Dr. Emerson, 1987.

Louis XIV's imposition of the horizontal birth position reported in Joseph Chilton Pearce, *Magical Child* (New York: E.P. Dutton, 1977), pp. 48 and 234.

Pages 119–121: Marshall H. Klaus, John H. Kennell, and Phyllis H. Klaus, *Mothering the Mother: How a Doula Can Help You Have a Shorter, Easier, Healthier Birth* (Reading, MA: Addison-Wesley, 1993).

Epilogue

Page 128: Jean Liedloff, *The Continuum Concept* (New York: Addison Wesley, 1977).

Page 129: Rachel Naomi Remen, *Kitchen Table Wisdom* (New York: Berkeley Publishing, 1996), pp. 311–313.

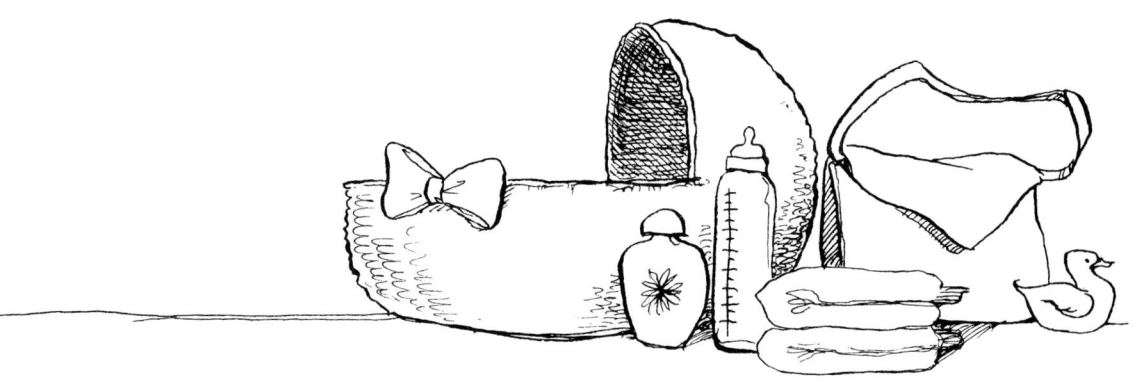

About the Authors
and
Resources for Further Growth

William R. Emerson, Ph.D., is a teacher, writer, and leader in the field of birth psychology. He has been named an honorary fellow by the National Institute of Mental Health for his scholarly excellence and his contributions to the field of psychology. For more than thirty years, he has been a pioneer in treatment methods for healing birth trauma in infants and children. He is also a renowned expert in treatment methods for adults and is recognized worldwide for his contributions. He is a frequent speaker at psychology conferences, is a radio and television personality, and conducts treatment and training seminars throughout the United States and Europe.

For anyone who wishes to follow up this book by seeking psychotherapy, training or other resources, please contact:
Dennis, Sheila & Matt Linn
Phone & Fax: (970) 476-9235
E-mail: dsjlinn@aol.com

Dr. Emerson has helped compile a list of referral sources for those who would like to receive professional treatment for prenatal and perinatal trauma for themselves or their children. To obtain a copy, please contact: APPPAH, Box 994, Geyserville, CA 95441, tel. (707) 857-4041, fax (707) 857-4042, web site www.birth psychology.com.

Dennis, Sheila, and Matt Linn work together as a team, integrating physical, emotional, and spiritual wholeness. They have worked as hospital chaplains and therapists and currently as retreat leaders and spiritual companions. They have taught courses on processes for healing in more than forty countries and in many universities and hospitals, including a course for doctors accredited by the American Medical Association. Dennis and Sheila live in Colorado with their son, John. Matt lives in a Jesuit community in Minnesota.

The Linns are the authors of seventeen books, including *Healing of Memories, Healing Life's Hurts, Healing the Dying, Praying With Another for Healing, Healing the Greatest Hurt, Healing the Eight Stages of Life, Belonging, Good Goats, Healing Spiritual Abuse & Religious Addiction, Sleeping With Bread, Don't Forgive Too Soon, Simple Ways To Pray for Healing* and *Healing the Purpose of Your Life*, all published by Paulist Press. These books have sold more than a million copies in English and have been translated into more than fifteen languages, including Spanish. Most are accompanied by audio and videotapes that can be used as courses in a wide variety of settings, such as parishes, prisons, 12-Step recovery groups, and psychotherapy groups. Videotapes can be borrowed on a donation basis by those who cannot afford to purchase them. For a complete list of materials and for a schedule of retreats and conferences, please contact: Re-Member Ministries, 3914-A Michigan Ave., St. Louis, MO 63118, tel. (314) 865-0729 or (970) 476-9235, fax (314) 773-3115 or (970) 476-9235.